Smoothies
for
Kidneys

- No-Nonsense Approach to Food and Kidney Function
- Smoothies to Prevent or Slow Kidney Damage
- Smoothies for All Kidney Disease Stages, Even Dialysis

Victoria L. Hulett, J.D.
Kidney Transplant Recipient

Jennifer L. Waybright, R.N.
Kidney Donor and Nurse

Smoothies for Kidneys

Copyright 2014 by KidneySteps, LLC

This book contains research findings as interpreted by the authors and the opinions and ideas of the authors. It is intended to provide helpful and informative material relating to kidney disease. It is sold with the understanding that the authors and publishers are not medical doctors. The reader should consult his/her healthcare provider before adopting suggestions in this book.

Authors and publisher specifically disclaim all responsibility for any liability, loss, or risk, personal or otherwise, incurred as a consequence, directly or indirectly, of use and application of any contents of this book.

All rights reserved. No part of this publication may be reproduced, stored in a retrieval system, or transmitted by any means—electronic, mechanical, photographic, photocopying, recording, or otherwise—without written permission from the authors.

ISBN-13:978-1495232176
ISBN-10:1495232174

Printed in the United States of America.
Order more copies at: www.kidneysteps.com

Acknowledgements

We very much appreciate the willingness of the following medical professionals who provided important review of sections of this book:

- Brandy Jones, R.D., C.D. Ms. Jones works with kidney and dialysis patients as a renal dietitian at a leading Midwest transplant center. We sincerely appreciate her particular focus on the smoothie recipes in Parts 5 and 6 of the book.
- Tim E. Taber, M.D., FACP. Dr. Taber is a leading nephrologist and authority on kidney health, disease, and treatments. Dr. Taber practices and teaches at Indiana University Health, Indianapolis, Indiana. We deeply appreciate his review of substantive sections of this book.

We extend deepest thanks to Deborah Carrithers, Indianapolis, Indiana for her patience and creativity in formatting this book and providing valuable suggestions in style.

Many thanks to our smoothie testers who provided critical opinions about taste, texture, color, and the mouth feel of each smoothie. Adult and child testers included:

- Sarah Almy, accounting student, San Marcos, Texas.
- Jack Drockelman, age 9, "The Smoothie Kid," Seabrook Island, South Carolina.
- Molly Hulett, writer, Seabrook Island, South Carolina.
- Robert Hulett, lawyer, Indianapolis, Indiana
- Amy Kemper, contributor to kidneysteps.com, Indianapolis, Indiana.
- Christopher (Kit) Kemper, administrator of kidneysteps.com, Indianapolis, Indiana.
- Sullivan Kemper, age 4, Indianapolis, Indiana.
- Nicole Kierein, PhD, Newton, Massachusetts.
- Clara Skendzel, age 4, Newton, Massachusetts.
- Eva Skendzel, age 8, Newton, Massachusetts.
- Benjamin D. Waybright, age 13, smoothie creator and daily smoothie drinker, Carmel, Indiana.
- Spencer T. Waybright, age 10, Carmel, Indiana.

VLH and *JLW*

Contents

Introduction Why Us? i

Part 1 Kidney Smarts 1

Chapter 1: Respect Those Beans 3

   Kidneys: Little Workhorses 3
   Chronic Kidney Disease 101 5
   Kidneys and Heart: Partners in Distress 8

Chapter 2: Kidney Disease:
          Often Food-Based 11

   Diabetes: Diet-Driven in Most 11
   High Blood Pressure: Help It Head South 13
   The Spare-Tire: Separate Creature 15
   Sugar: Not So Sweet for Kidney Health 17
   Fats: The Good, the Bad, the Ugly 20
   Setting Our Kids Up for CKD 23

Part 2 Smoothies and Health 27

Chapter 3: Eats Kidneys Love 29

   DASH for Health 29
   Renal Diet: A Confusing Label 31
   Antioxidants: Health Superheroes 32
   Phytochemicals: Keys to Better Health 34
   Fiber: Disease Fighter 35

Chapter 4: Slowing Kidney Damage with Produce........ 39

Acidosis: Internal Burn.................................... 39
Inflammation: Internal Attack........................... 42
Uric Acid: Contributes to Acidosis...................... 43
Be Protein-Picky.. 44
Those Pesky Electrolytes.................................. 47
Food After a Kidney Transplant......................... 54

Chapter 5: Top Kidney Protection Tips.......... 59

Part 3 | Smoothie Basics......... 63

Chapter 6: Kidney-Health Smoothie Tips....... 65

Ignore "All Natural" Claims............................. 65
Juicing.. 66
Organic versus Conventional........................... 67
Caution with Dietary Supplements.................... 68
Blender Layering... 72

Chapter 7: "Why Smoothies?" Wrap-Up......... 73

Part 4 | Smoothies for Most........ 79

Part 5 | Smoothies with Reduced K and P...... 127

Part 6 | Smoothies for Dialysis... 145

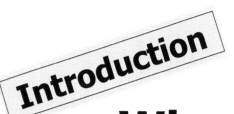

Why *Us*?

Vicki's Story:

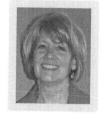

Learning you have a progressive disease is devastating. I vividly recall the day my family doctor told me I had lost nearly 70 percent of my kidney function. A nephrologist later diagnosed my condition as chronic kidney disease (CKD). After genetic testing, we learned the cause was Alport Syndrome, an inherited defect that can leave its victim blind, deaf, and without kidney function.

While not then identified as "Alport," the same genetic disease likely killed my mother and several others in her bloodline. The nephrologist said I would face dialysis within three years. My sister also learned she had Alport, as did all three of her daughters.

I researched frantically in hopes of finding ways to reverse this damnable kidney disease, not then knowing that Alport can't be reversed. It has its own genetic timeline of progression. While drugs lowered my resulting blood pressure, no drug slowed progression of my CKD. Successive blood and urine tests showed worsening kidney function.

The only hopes offered in research were diet and exercise, factors within my control in a disease that leaves one out of control. I routinely exercised, but I geared up my efforts. Exercise did help relieve my fatigue and melancholy feelings.

As to diet, I knew the basics and was already a developing vegetarian, but this was after years of abusing my body with the "standard American diet" (SAD). You know that eating pattern: red and processed meats, fast food, daily colas, sugary desserts, salty restaurant food, fatty snacks. Some of those bad habits snuck into my good-eating attempts. So, I dug in my heels and threw out any remaining junk in the house, stopped eating out so often, and avoided processed foods.

While diet and exercise changes did not stop my CKD, they did slow its progression. My "three years to dialysis" doubled to six. Moreover, I felt good despite worsening kidney function, and I never needed to alter my diet to reduce potassium or phosphorus, despite my high intake of fruits, vegetables, nuts, and low-fat dairy. Most important, my cardiovascular system remained strong and without the customary defects that develop in so many kidney patients.

I continued working full-time as an attorney, and no one guessed I had CKD, even as I entered stage 5 and was told to prepare for dialysis. My external health appeared normal; I had no nausea or loss of appetite; my weight remained steady; and I retained amazing energy.

I never did prepare for dialysis. My angel of a daughter decided I should have one of her kidneys. With both a heavy heart and a joyous one, I eventually accepted it. I can never repay Jennifer for her loving generosity.

The day before transplant surgery, I worked 10 hours, exercised, and enjoyed a hearty meal with a glass of wine. Transplant surgery went without a hitch, and my daughter and I were both released from the hospital a couple of days later. Within two weeks, we were both back full-time.

My nephrologist summed it up pretty well when he said: "Your diet and other lifestyle habits gave you an edge most kidney patients don't have. Most of them are quite ill, and you avoided that suffering."

Jennifer's Turn:

I am a rarity in our family (mother's side) because I did not inherit Alport Syndrome but grew up with two perfectly healthy organs. I am also the only nurse in the family.

What really makes me a rarity, though, is that I donated my left kidney to my mother 5 years ago. She initially refused my offer of a kidney, but I left her little option. While she may be the lawyer, I'm pretty clever myself. I worked with the transplant center in our hometown to offer my kidney to any matching person in need. The transplant center notified Mom. What could she do but accept my donation, which is where I wanted my kidney to go. I knew she would take careful care of it by following healthful diet and exercise habits and adhering to lab and drug requirements.

While donating was the best decision I ever made, it does leave me with a single kidney that I carefully protect. As a nurse and because of my kidney donation, I stay alert to newly-released kidney studies, including research linking diet to kidney health. Diet is within our control, which I like. Each time we put a food item to our lips, we make a choice to consume something that will promote health or is destined to harm it.

Most patients I see at the hospital where I work have unknowingly abused their kidneys, as well as their bodies, with lousy lifestyle habits, particularly poor food choices. The results are not pretty, and often the patient has no idea how to go about changing dietary habits.

I've discovered that controlling what we put in our mouths is likely the most important step in protecting and improving kidney health. Even people who have no remaining kidney function and are on dialysis can improve their heart health with sound food selections. Cardiovascular disease is the primary killer of kidney patients.

We want to share with you what we've learned about food and kidney health. We've designed each smoothie with kidney and heart health as priorities. I enjoy these smoothies and drink them daily. It's so convenient to whirl one in my handy dandy, single-serve blender and drink it as I rush to work or to take one of my two sons to sports or band practice. My boys love smoothies, too.

Please use this book to learn and enjoy.

We wish you kidney health!

Part 1
Kidney *Smarts*

Most people don't realize how important kidneys are to overall health until those tiny organs are in crisis. Kidneys do much more than make urine. They help control blood pressure, stimulate red blood cell production, maintain the stability and purity of our internal environment, and participate in bone formation.

An estimated 6 out of 10 Americans will develop kidney disease over their lifetimes, driven primarily by rising rates of diabetes, obesity, hypertension, and cardiovascular disease. Each of these kidney-damaging causes largely results from poor diet: too much sugary, fatty, salty, and processed food. The good news is that you can do something about that. So, let's begin now.

CHAPTER 1: RESPECT THOSE BEANS

Kidneys: Little Workhorses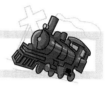

Kidneys deserve respect! These 6-ounce, fist-sized, bean-shaped organs work 24/7 to perform their three main jobs:

🫘 Remove Wastes

Kidneys filter an amazing 200 liters of blood each day to remove toxic waste products and excess water, which become urine. The urine continuously trickles down a ureter leading from each kidney to collect in the **bladder**.

The filtering units in the kidneys are called **nephrons**, and each kidney has over 1 million of them. Nephrons encase a clump of the tiniest of blood vessels, or capillaries, that do the actual filtering. Each clump is known as a **glomerulus** (the plural is **glomeruli**).

The covering of each glomerulus is semi-permeable, with tiny holes that act like a coffee filter, to allow small molecules (extra water and waste products) to move out of the blood flowing through the kidney and to prevent larger molecules of substances still needed by the body from escaping.

Blood pressure in glomeruli is higher than in other vessels of the body to assist in pushing out the wastes dissolved in the blood. This higher pressure makes the glomeruli vulnerable to hypertension. If you don't control high blood pressure, it eventually ruptures the glomeruli, destroying them and leading to kidney disease.

The wastes being removed by the kidneys are normal by-products of your cells as they convert food to energy for all of your body's activities. Wastes include nitrogen-containing products, such as **urea**, toxic to the body. So, removal of these toxins is important for survival.

⬤ Regulate Chemicals

An extremely important function of kidneys is to maintain a constant level of certain vital chemicals in your blood, such as sodium, calcium, potassium, phosphorus, water, and acid/base. Kidneys do this by filtering out excess amounts of these chemicals accumulating from your diet. When kidneys fail to function properly, excesses build in the blood, which can result in death. That is why you must adjust your diet in advanced kidney disease to limit consumption of foods containing large amounts of the chemicals the kidneys can no longer adequately filter and balance.

⬤ Release Hormones

Kidneys act as glands, secreting hormones to control blood pressure, produce red blood cells, and stimulate bone growth. The hormone impacting blood pressure is **renin**. Kidneys monitor blood pressure as blood flows through them. If pressure is too low, kidneys release renin to prompt a chain of reactions that raise pressure. If kidneys aren't functioning properly, they release too much renin, resulting in the high blood pressure so common in kidney disease.

Kidneys also release **erythropoietin** (EPO) to stimulate bone marrow to produce red blood cells. EPO production declines when kidneys are damaged, which explains why **anemia** (not enough red blood cells) is common in kidney disease.

Finally, those amazing kidneys convert the form of vitamin D you obtain from exposure to sun or from food to a form the body can use. That active form of vitamin D is **calcitriol**, and it stimulates the intestines to absorb calcium and phosphorus from food for bone growth and other critical cell functions. When kidneys fail, they can't make adequate calcitriol, no matter how much sun you get or how many vitamin D pills you pop. Hence, vitamin D deficiency and weakened bones are common features in kidney disease.

Chronic Kidney Disease 101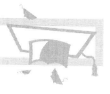

Staggering Numbers

Over 26 million U.S. adults and thousands of children have **chronic kidney disease (CKD)**.[1] Over half of the U.S. may develop CKD thanks to rising rates of diabetes, hypertension, and obesity.

> Recent research indicates Americans have a lifetime CKD risk of 59.1 percent.[2]

Amazingly, over 90 percent of individuals with CKD are not aware of it, often until after the disease has progressed to the point where the person is very ill.[3] CKD develops slowly and silently, over time. Most CKD cases result from diabetes (leading cause of CKD), hypertension (second leading cause), obesity, cardiovascular disease, or overuse of kidney-toxic drugs (such as anti-inflammatories).[4] In nearly all of these cases, CKD was lifestyle-triggered – poor diet, lack of exercise, failure to control weight – and potentially preventable.

Once a person has CKD, it is rarely reversible. However, detecting the disease early allows intervention with medication, dietary changes, and weight loss to slow or even stop CKD progression and avoid **kidney failure**, also known as **end-stage renal disease (ESRD)**, where dialysis or a kidney transplant is needed.

Diagnosing CKD

The National Kidney Foundation (NKF) recommends simple blood and urine tests to determine CKD. These tests reveal whether, and to what extent, kidneys are leaking a type of protein called **albumin** into the urine, and the stage of CKD, determined by **estimated glomerular filtration rate** or **GFR**.[5]

Protein consistently appearing in urine (termed **proteinuria** or **albuminuria**) is not a good sign. Working kidneys normally keep protein in the body rather than letting it leak into urine.

Proteinuria is an early indication of kidney damage. Having even small amounts of proteinuria also means an increased risk for cardiovascular disease, says the NKF.[6] Proteinuria is also strongly linked to mortality.

> In a study of over 810,000 patients, proteinuria was tied to shorter life spans of between 8.2 years (mild proteinuria) to 17.4 years (heavy proteinuria).[7]

You can check your own urine for protein by dipping a protein test strip (get them online or from a pharmacist) into your clean urine. Color changes mean protein.

GFR is an estimate of total kidney function. It is the rate at which all of your glomeruli are working to filter your blood. GFR is always an estimate and will vary somewhat from test to test, but usually not dramatically. The higher the GFR, the better the kidneys function.

CKD is classified into stages 1-5, based on GFR. The early stages 1 and 2 usually require the presence of kidney damage such as proteinuria, along with reduced GFR to be CKD.[8] *See* Appendix 1 for the NKF's new chart of the stages of CKD as determined by a range of GFR and albuminuria measurements.

> If you have CKD, you will hear the word **creatinine**. Creatinine is a waste product created from the normal metabolism of a protein called creatinine as muscles burn energy. The level of creatinine in the blood normally stays stable because working kidneys only filter out excess. If kidneys are not working properly, they allow too much creatinine to stay in the blood. Creatinine is not a perfect measure of kidney function, but it is used.

Many clinicians describe moderate CKD as stage 3 because having a GFR of 60 or less represents a loss of about 50 percent of kidney function. Ample evidence tells us, though, that CKD significantly raises risk of cardiovascular issues and results in destructive chemical imbalances even in earlier stages. [9] So, being aggressive in care and diet at any CKD stage is important.

Measure of Kidney Function

Stage One GFR 90 or above

Estimated GFR of 90 or above is considered normal. However, some people, even with normal GFR, have other signs of possible kidney damage, such as protein or blood in the urine.

Stage Two GFR 60 to 89

Stage Two is kidney damage with a mild decrease in GFR. Glomeruli show damage, and small amounts of blood and/or protein usually leak into the urine. With good control over blood pressure and blood glucose levels, individuals might remain in Stage Two.

Stage Three GFR 30 to 59

Stage Three is considered moderate kidney disease. When a patient presents GFR of less than 60 for 3 or more months, the patient is diagnosed with CKD. When CKD has advanced to this stage, signs of bone deterioration, heart and vessel disease, and anemia are common.

Stage Four GFR 15 to 29

Stage Four constitutes severe CKD. Large amounts of protein may leak into the urine and high blood pressure usually exists. Cardiovascular issues are common, as are anemia and chemical imbalances requiring diet modifications and drug intervention. During Stage Four, the patient considers dialysis or kidney transplantation options.

Stage Five GFR less than 15

Stage Five is end-stage renal disease (ESRD). Kidneys do not work well enough to keep the patient alive for long without dialysis or a transplant.

Aging and Kidneys

Despite declarations from octogenarians that our later decades are better, the kidneys may not agree. Aging is tough on kidneys, and kidney function normally declines beginning at about age 30. GFR decreases by as much as 7 percent per decade, so that by age 60, we only have 75 percent of our former kidney function. Kidneys also shrink in size, just as the aging body does, which affects function. [10]

However, just because kidney function and size decline with age does not necessarily mean kidney disease. A diagnosis of CKD is based on GFR slipping to 60 or under. The presence of protein in urine increases the likelihood of CKD.

Age-related changes in kidneys make them more susceptible to impact from diabetes, hypertension, and other CKD-triggering conditions. That's why CKD is more prevalent in older people then in younger ones, and more dialysis patients are over 60 than under. [11] Diets high in fruits and vegetables and exercise are shown to help preserve kidney function in older folks. [12]

Kidneys & Heart: Partners in Disease

Quiz: If you have kidney disease, are you more likely to die from kidney disease or heart disease?
Answer: Bingo, if you answered, "heart disease."

On top of other woes accompanying kidney disease, people with deteriorating kidney function are likely to develop heart and vessel problems.[1] Kidney patients are at high risk for cardiovascular disease.[2]

Kidney and heart health are intimately tied, bonded like brothers. When one of these organs suffers, so does the other. The tie is related to the heart-damaging chemical imbalances and waste buildup resulting from faulty kidney function.[3] Recent speculation is that these conditions damage the lining of blood vessels throughout the body, resulting in cardiovascular disease.[4]

Did you ever wonder why only about 800,000 of the 26+ million Americans with CKD advance to stage 5 or end stage, where dialysis or a kidney transplant is required to continue to live? Part of the reason is that even in the early stages of CKD, patients are more likely to develop cardio-vascular disease and die from it than progress to stage 5.[5] Once in stage 5, life still ends primarily because of heart events.[6]

> **Life's Simple 7:**
> 1. No smoking
> 2. Be physically active
> 3. Follow a healthy diet (more on this later)
> 4. Have a normal weight
> 5. Maintain low blood sugar
> 6. Maintain low blood pressure
> 7. Maintain low cholesterol

The good news is that you can lower your cardiovascular risks. Because the heart and kidneys are so intertwined, a heart-healthy lifestyle becomes a kidney-healthy lifestyle.[7] In fact, people with heart-healthy habits can live longer and better, despite CKD.[8]

The American Heart Association identifies seven primary lifestyle factors to help keep your ticker (and kidneys) in top shape. These factors are **Life's Simple 7**.[9] See the box above.

While we can't yank that cigarette out of your otherwise lovely lips or strap those comfy shoes on your pods for that daily 30-minute brisk walk, we can arm you with a delicious variety of healthy smoothies to help you meet the 5 remaining lifestyle factors. Now, that is good news.

By increasing your intake of heart-healthy foods and moving away from the standard American diet (SAD), you might improve your health status and live longer, even if you already have heart problems. Fatty, salty, sugary, processed SAD food harms your vessels, including the ones in your kidneys.[10]

Substitute one or two of these kidney and heart healthy drinkables each day for that bacon breakfast, hamburger and fries lunch, or pizza dinner. With conscientiousness, you could see your weight move toward desirable; your blood pressure, blood sugar, and cholesterol levels drop; your heart strengthen; and, perhaps, your kidney function improve.

CHAPTER 2:
KIDNEY DISEASE: OFTEN FOOD-BASED

Kidney disease has several causes. Some causes are genetic, some result from birth defects, and some arise from use of destructive medications. Nearly 80 percent of kidney disease cases, though, are lifestyle-based: eating too much of the wrong foods for too long.

Diabetes: Diet-Driven in Most

Diabetes is the leading cause of kidney disease and kidney failure (ESRD), and a whopping 26 million Americans are diabetic. An additional 79 million are pre-diabetic, and many prediabetics already show signs of kidney damage.[1] More than 40 percent of diabetics develop kidney disease, the majority within 10 years of their diabetes diagnosis.[2]

While it is possible to live a long and relatively healthy life with diabetes, once kidney disease develops, risk of dying prematurely skyrockets. A recent study found that people with both CKD and diabetes are 31 percent more likely to die within the 10-year study period compared to those not having both diseases.[3]

In diabetes, the pancreas either fails to make sufficient insulin (type 1 diabetes), or the body's cells ignore insulin (type 2 diabetes). Insulin is a hormone that transports glucose from our blood following a meal and into our cells where it is used for energy production.

Fewer than 10 percent of diabetes is type 1, which is not caused by diet and lifestyle and for which the only cure is a pancreas transplant. Nearly 30 percent of type 1 diabetics develop CKD.

The remaining 90+ percent of diabetes is type 2, caused primarily by indulging in inferior food choices. In type 2, the body's cells fail to respond correctly to insulin, a condition termed **insulin resistance,** which develops in pre-diabetes. Insulin resistance requires the pancreas to make extra insulin to keep blood glucose levels normal. Over time, the exhausted pancreas can't keep up with, or even respond to, the extra need for insulin caused by an over-consumption of poor quality calories. Diabetes is the reward.

Excess glucose in blood scars and inflames the tiny capillaries comprising the glomeruli (filtering units) of the kidneys. Damaged glomeruli also cause blood pressure to rise. Eventually, the filtering ability of the kidneys is destroyed. This form of CKD is known as **diabetic nephropathy.**

Over a third of diabetics with CKD don't know they have diabetes, let alone CKD:

> Researchers analyzed 8,200 U.S. adults and found that 42% of them with undiagnosed diabetes had CKD, as did 18% of pre-diabetics.[4]

So, these unaware souls continue with their same poor eating and exercise habits, getting fatter and worsening their diabetes and CKD. No wonder diabetes is the seventh leading cause of death in the U.S.[5]

Dialysis patients with diabetes (about half) have a boosted risk for heart attacks and strokes. The combination of ESRD and dialysis is particularly life-threatening. Depending on age, some of these folks have 12 times the risk of a cardiovascular death than if they only had one of the diseases.[6]

Sugar consumption is particularly threatening in both the making of a diabetic and after the disease exists. Consuming fructose in refined grains (white rice, white flour), processed foods, and sweetened beverages results quickly in elevated blood glucose levels. Sweetened drinks, a leading source of added sugar in the diet, are so damaging that the American Diabetes Association (ADA) recommends that people at risk for or with diabetes flat-out avoid them.[7] Even diet soda is harmful. Just one daily soda raises odds for diabetes:

> Study participants who drank one sugared soda daily had an 18% greater risk of developing diabetes. Two sodas raised diabetes risk to 36%. Two cans of diet soda increased diabetes risk by 52%. [8]

ADA research shows that the **DASH** (Dietary Approaches to Stop Hypertension) diet lowers blood sugar in people with type 2 diabetes (more on DASH later). Both the ADA and the NKF recommend the DASH diet in diabetes.[9] In fact, type 2 diabetes can be controlled and even reversed with a healthy diet and some exercise. Lowering blood glucose levels reduces risk of developing CKD or progressing to ESRD.

DASH emphasizes calorie control and eating unprocessed, non-refined, nutrient dense foods that keep glucose blood levels in check. Our DASH-friendly smoothies are perfect for those in fear of or with diabetes.

Yes, you can have the fruit in smoothies. Diabetics who enjoy adequate whole fruit (rather than juice) seem to shed more pounds and control blood sugar better than diabetics eating fewer than two pieces of fruit daily.[10] The carbohydrate restriction you've heard about for diabetes applies to empty, refined carbs—not to complex carbs found in fruits, vegetables, and whole grains, primary components of kidney-friendly smoothies.

High Blood Pressure: Help It Head South

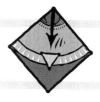

High blood pressure or **hypertension** is the second leading cause of CKD, accounting for about 25 percent of all cases.[1] If you already have kidney disease and don't have high blood pressure, odds are you soon will. Over 74 percent of younger CKD patients and 92 percent of older ones (age 65 and older) suffer from it.[2] These depressing blood pressure rates are much higher than the already-too-high 31 percent in the general U.S. adult population.[3]

If not treated and controlled, hypertension does more than cause kidney damage. It also leads to cardiovascular disease, including heart attacks and strokes. Just having high blood pressure substantially increases risk of early death.[4]

Unfortunately, blood pressure control is achieved in only about 26 percent of folks with early CKD. With such poor control, it is not surprising that hypertension is a leader in causing CKD to progress to kidney failure (ESRD) and dialysis – that is, if the person does not die first from heart failure or stroke, a too-common CKD event.[5]

The NKF recommends use of whatever therapy is necessary to keep blood pressure at or below 140/90 mm Hg in CKD patients with no albuminuria, including transplant recipients. A stricter target of 130/80 mm Hg applies to patients with albuminuria.[6] That limit applies to both the **systolic** (top number) and the **diastolic** (bottom number) readings. Unfolding research suggests the NKF's blood pressure guidelines may be too aggressive for older kidney patients, but speak with your doctor.

> AHA recommends an automatic cuff-style blood pressure monitor at home to measure your own pressure a couple of times daily.

In a study of 650,000 veterans with CKD from 2004 to 2006, those who kept systolic pressure at 140-159 mm Hg and diastolic pressure at 90-99 mm Hg had the lowest mortality rates compared to those with normal blood pressure (less than 120/80 mm Hg).[7]

As to medication, most kidney patients not on dialysis will take an angiotensin converting enzyme (ACE) inhibitor, angiotensin receptor blocker (ARB), or renin inhibitor to control blood pressure. These classes of drugs are shown to help preserve kidney function, as well as lower proteinuria.[8]

Besides medication, lifestyle changes can reduce risk of high blood pressure by up to 80 percent, shows research.[9] In particular, a diet high in potassium-rich and nitrate-rich fruits and vegetables lowers blood pressure and cardiovascular risk.[10] The AHA and the American Society of Hypertension recommend the following lifestyle changes, beginning with a high-produce diet, for blood pressure control:

- ✓ Eat a DASH-like diet (here we go with DASH, again)
- ✓ Maintain a healthy weight
- ✓ Exercise regularly
- ✓ Don't smoke
- ✓ Limit alcohol
- ✓ Limit painkiller use

The DASH diet was specifically designed to lower blood pressure. You truly can eat to lower blood pressure. The fruits, vegetables, whole grains, and nuts/seeds you'll see in the DASH-based smoothies are tailored to contribute to improved health, including blood pressure health. Replace a salty breakfast of processed meats (bacon, sausage, ham) with a nutritious smoothie to begin your day of blood pressure control.

The Spare Tire: Separate Creature

Obesity

Thanks to a rapidly worsening diet of fizzy drinks and cheap fast food, nearly 70 percent of us are overweight, and half of the overweight are obese.[1] **Obesity** is now an official disease. Sadly, almost 20 percent of our children are also obese, unheard of just 30 years ago.

Obesity leads to kidney disease and contributes to a number of other serious medical conditions, including cardiovascular disease, hypertension, type 2 diabetes, cancer. In fact, all of these diseases are more common in overweight and obese people than in normal-weight people.[2] Currently, one in five Americans dies from obesity.[3]

Obese individuals, particularly the so-called "apple-shaped" who carry more fat around their bellies than their hips, have a much higher risk for developing kidney disease than normal-weight and pear-shaped folks. The bigger the person is, the greater the risks for proteinuria and CKD.

> A recent study of 315 adults found that a higher waist-to-hip ratio and being overweight elevated CKD risk. Each unit increase in waist-to-hip measure lowered GFR as if the kidneys had aged 4 years. [4]

Kidney disease also progresses to end-stage faster in the obese. The obese propel to dialysis at twice the speed of their thinner counterparts.[5]

It's that visceral fat, the fat cascading over the belt and dangerously wrapping around internal organs (particularly the liver), that's the problem. Visceral fat acts like a separate creature with a life of its own. It is metabolically active, spewing out disease-generating chemicals and causing dangerous internal inflammation. Waist fat has long been associated with cardio-vascular events and death in CKD. [6]

Poor diet may change the mix of microbes in the gut to obesity-promoting microbes. [7] Yikes!

The only cure for the visceral fat creature is to lose it, which is easier said than done. However, weight loss provides an avenue to slow, halt, and in some cases, reverse kidney disease. A great way to begin losing weight is by giving up those sweet colas, perhaps exchanging them for sweet-tasting smoothies. You can make a guilt-free, weight-loss-promoting smoothie in five little minutes.

Metabolic Syndrome

Obesity is tied to **metabolic syndrome**, which is present in one out of four American adults. If you have three of the following five features, you have the syndrome.

	Metabolic Syndrome[8]	
	Women	Men
Waist Size	More than 35-inch waist	More than 40-inch waist
Triglycerides	150 or higher	150 or higher
HDL ("good" cholesterol)	Under 50	Under 40
Blood Pressure Systolic Diastolic	130 or higher 85 or higher	130 or higher 85 or higher
Blood Sugar	110 or higher	110 or higher

Metabolic syndrome results from an inability of the body to process fats and sugars, almost always because we eat too much of the stuff and exercise too little. Metabolic syndrome is a sign of insulin resistance and substantially raises risks for type 2 diabetes, heart disease, mortality, nonfatty liver disease, cancer, gout, and CKD.[9]

Besides being strongly associated with the development and progression of CKD, metabolic syndrome also seems to raise the already very high risk of cardiovascular death in kidney patients.[10] However, metabolic syndrome doesn't have to be a one-way street to chronic disease. Consuming a healthy diet of mostly plant-based foods and cutting back on red meat, refined grains, sugary drinks, and salty snacks can reverse metabolic syndrome.[11] Why not begin with a daily smoothie?

Sugar: Not So Sweet for Health

As trans fatty acids disappear from our foods, **added sugars** are stepping in as the most dangerous single food we consume. Unlike trans fats, though, sugar also appears addictive.[1] We are learning that **fructose** in sugar is the real health villain, especially given the quantities Americans consume in sweetened beverages and processed, packaged foods.

Each American slams down 63 pounds of concentrated fructose each year, and 70 percent of it comes from sweetened beverages, estimates the USDA.[2] We seem to crave our soft drinks, sports drinks, fruit drinks, punches, sweetened coffee and tea drinks, and energy drinks spiked with added sweeteners. A cola is about 65 percent fructose!

Fructose accounts for half the molecules in sucrose, which is table sugar. The other portion is glucose. Glucose does not taste sweet like fructose, and our cells use glucose for energy. We ordinarily handle glucose well, assuming we don't overeat and we retain the natural ability to control blood levels of glucose with insulin.[3]

Fructose is found in fruit, but whole fruit also contains fiber and numerous nutrients, making whole fruit a great food choice. It's when the fiber is removed by turning the fruit into juice, that fructose can have adverse metabolic effects.

SUGAR BY OTHER NAMES:
Most sugar by any name contains around 50 percent fructose. Corn syrup and lactose (the natural sugar in milk) do not.
SOME SUGARS TO LIMIT:
Beet sugar, brown sugar, cane juice, maple syrup, molasses, raw sugar, rice syrup, table sugar, juices from concentrate (e.g., orange, grape, but apple contains 67 percent fructose), high fructose corn syrup, agave (88 percent fructose), sugar alcohol.

Food manufactures have concocted a concentrated, fiberless form of fructose, **high fructose corn syrup**, that is low in cost and acts as a preservative for a long shelf life. This form of fructose is used in nearly all sweetened drinks and processed foods.

It's no surprise that consumption of fructose has increased nearly 2,000 percent over the past three decades, along with the epidemics of obesity, diabetes, metabolic syndrome, hypertension, cancer, and kidney disease.[4]

Kidney-Damaging

Most research regarding the harmful effects of fructose use sweetened beverages because nearly three-fourths of our fructose intake comes from them. Colas are linked to elevated uric acid and creatinine levels. One startling study found that just two glasses of cola per day doubled risk of CKD.[5] Colas also increase odds of developing kidney stones.[6]

Added sugars, whether as fructose or in other forms, can harm kidney function, raise uric acid levels, and create damaging internal inflammation. Added sugar may well be the cause of many kidney diseases, concluded a recent study.[7] In contrast, diets low in added sugar result in a reduced risk of CKD and in lowered blood pressure and inflammation in people who already have CKD.[8]

Diabetes-Causing and Heart-Damaging

Swigging six and a half sugar-sweetened drinks per week doubles risk for diabetes, elevates blood pressure, and raises risk of heart attack and stroke.[9] You'll recall that diabetes is the leading cause of CKD and of end-stage renal disease.

Unlike glucose, which our cells metabolize, fructose is metabolized by the liver, a more difficult process. The liver can't process the excessive amounts of fructose often consumed and converts it to fat. Some of the fat is stored in the liver and some goes into the bloodstream.

As excessive fructose intake continues, the liver becomes fatty, which causes insulin resistance. The fat that the liver dumps into the bloodstream raises triglycerides and LDLs (both bad) as well as heart disease risk. The fat also collects in the belly as dangerous, disease-causing visceral fat that leads to metabolic syndrome, obesity, and other diseases. Added sugars also appear to boost artery disease and increase cholesterol levels.[10]

Obesity

Clearly, too many calories from anything–sugary beverages, beer, burgers, pizza, fries, ice cream, or dozens of other foods–explains Americans' serious weight epidemic. But it's now becoming apparent that calories from added sugars are more likely than other calories to head for the waist and result in obesity.

No one denies that sugary beverages can plaster on pounds, and half the population drinks 1 to 2 liters each day![11] Studies find that sweetened pop drinkers gain weight, and it's likely to be around the belly as dangerous visceral fat.[12] Fructose in most added sugars appears to boost fat content in liver, muscle, and the gut. The result of continued excess consumption of fructose and other calories is obesity and most other chronic diseases.

> The Nutritional Facts panel on a food item tells you how many grams of added sugars are in a serving. Multiply the grams by 4 to get calories of sugar. Divide by 4 to get teaspoons.

In a national survey of more than 16,000 people, roughly 78 percent of women and 67 percent of men consumed too much added sugar.[13] The American Heart Association recommends that women get no more than 100 calories of added sugars per day (25 grams, about 6 teaspoons). A regular soft drink contains 8 teaspoons of added sugars. The recommendation for men is no more than 150 calories per day (37.5 grams, 9 teaspoons).[14]

Don't think you get a free pass by switching to artificial sweeteners. The latest research slams the fake stuff as confusing the body on how to respond to real sugar when it gets it, resulting in the body's failure to release insulin appropriately. Thus, up go blood sugar levels and blood pressure.[15]

We avoid added sugars and artificial sweeteners in nearly all these kidney-loving, health-promoting smoothies. Naturally sweet fruit does not need offensive added sugar.

Fats: The Good, The Bad, The Ugly

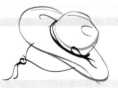

High **cholesterol** is common in kidney disease and can worsen kidney disease progression. The latest news is that high cholesterol may be tied, in part, to our heavy consumption of added sugars.[1]

Cholesterol is a waxy, fat-like substance the body uses for various cell functions and to make bile acids, hormones, vitamin D, and other essential chemicals. Your liver manufactures all the cholesterol you need.

Extra cholesterol from fatty and sugary foods accumulates in artery walls, forming plaque. Plaque narrows blood vessels, making them less flexible, a condition called **atherosclerosis** or hardening of the arteries. Plaque build-up in the arteries of the heart results in coronary artery disease, which plagues too many individuals with CKD. Plaque build-up in the tiny vessels of glomeruli destroys them, leading to or worsening CKD.

Fatty cholesterol and blood, like oil and water, do not mix. So, cholesterol travels through your bloodstream in packets called **lipoproteins**, with proteins on the outside and the cholesterol inside. A blood test for lipids usually measures two types of lipoproteins:

- ✓ **Low density lipoprotein**, or **LDL**, is bad cholesterol that carries fatty cholesterol to your body tissues. Most cholesterol in your blood is LDL.
- ✓ **High density lipoprotein,** or **HDL,** is good cholesterol that carries cholesterol away from your tissues to the liver for removal.

The most common fats in our system are **triglycerides,** which are made up of mostly **saturated fatty acids** and some **unsaturated fatty acids**. Saturated fats are important for numerous cell functions, but the body makes enough and doesn't need extra from foods. Extra raises unhealthy LDLs. Saturated fats are prevalent in red meat, whole milk, butter, cheese, ice cream, and many junk foods.

Unsaturated fats are classified as either **mono- or polyunsaturated** and are the reason that not all fats are bad. Monounsaturated fats (found in olive oil, nuts, fish, and avocados, for example) help lower blood levels of LDLs and triglycerides, cutting risk of stroke and heart disease.

Polyunsaturated fats consist of two major groups: **omega-3 fatty acids** (found in fish oils, nuts, seeds) and **omega-6 fatty**

acids (found in vegetable oils, such as canola, sunflower, and corn). Omega-3's are linked to a wide range of health benefits. Omega-6's are controversial, and some studies suggest they have inflammatory effects if not balanced with omega-3's.

A blood test is used to determine your lipid levels.

Lipids and Levels

Type of Lipid	Normal Level	Borderline High	Undesirable
Total Cholesterol	Less than 200	200-239	above 239
Low-density lipoprotein (LDL)(bad)	Less than 100	130-159	160-189 or above
High-density lipoprotein (HDL)(good)	Above 40 (60 or above is great!)	35-39	below 35
Triglycerides	Below 150	151-199	above 200

Having excess lipids in the blood is termed **hyperlipidemia**. A big cause of hyperlipidemia is fructose, and Americans pound down way too much of it. Study participants who consumed diets high in fructose (which is added to nearly all commercially-prepared products and beverages) had increased levels of LDLs and triglycerides after only two weeks.[2]

Hyperlipidemia is common in patients with CKD.[3] It is not only a risk factor for cardiovascular disease, but also seems to hasten progression of kidney disease.[4]

The jury is still out on whether taking cholesterol-lowering drugs—statins—slows progression of CKD. A large analysis found that taking statins slowed CKD progression somewhat.[5] However, researchers conclude that the possibility of death from cardiovascular disease is a significant threat in CKD, and statins reduce that risk. It remains unclear whether statins decrease mortality in dialysis patients.[6]

> ### Simple Rules for Lowering Cholesterol

Limit saturated fats (whole-fat dairy and red meat) because they kick your body's production of cholesterol into overdrive.

Avoid trans fat. Trans fat, another manufactured, cheap substance formed by partially hydrogenating vegetable oil, is always bad. Consuming trans fat increases bad LDL cholesterol, lowers good HDL cholesterol, and is linked to heart disease. While trans fat consumption has declined since 2006, you'll still find it in some margarines and baked goods (pie crust, pastries). So check the list of ingredients for "partially hydrogenated vegetable oil."

Avoid added sugars. Fructose is added to nearly all packaged and processed foods, whether or not they taste sweet, and to all sweetened beverages. Eliminate soft drinks and check all food labels for sugar.

Increase fiber. Soluble fiber in particular binds with cholesterol and helps carry it out of your system. A diet high in the ingredients found in our smoothies—fruits, vegetable, whole grains, nuts, and beans—provides that fiber.

Lose weight and exercise. We know, *yuck*—but important.

In the war against heart and kidney-damaging high cholesterol, substituting meals of pizza, burgers, fries, shakes, and colas for delicious, nutritious smoothies on a regular basis is a promising weapon to lower bad cholesterol and raise good HDLs.

Setting Our Kids Up for CKD

Little is more heart-wrenching than an infant or toddler stricken with CKD. The disease is devastating in every respect, its impact harsher in children than in older individuals. Young children with CKD nearly always inherited the disease, or it arose from a congenital defect. No one is to blame. The only good news is that over 40 percent of these children receive a kidney for transplantation within a year of listing.[1]

The remainder of this section is not about these children. Rather, it concerns the kids who are predestined to develop CKD and other serious diseases later in life, largely because of early dietary patterns. Patterns they unfortunately learn at home.

The percentage of our youth developing diabetes and obesity keeps growing. The latest data show that one-third of kids are overweight or obese.[2] Obesity in children is three times the rate it was just a generation ago. Diabetes in our young has increased over 22 percent in the last decade.[3]

What's worse, kids with obesity or type 2 diabetes end up with more health complications as adults and suffer those complications earlier in their lives than if they had reached adulthood before becoming obese or diabetic.[4] For example, obese and diabetic children are developing high blood pressure, normally an older adult issue, at unusually young ages.[5] In children hospitalized for hypertension, some are as young as two.[6] Children already have high cholesterol, atherosclerosis, and cardiac issues.[7] Sad!

Obviously, obesity, diabetes, and hypertension set these children up for kidney disease. No wonder new research tells us that over half of the U.S. may develop CKD during their lives.[8]

> In a recent study of 1.2 million 17-year-olds, those who were obese had 19 times the risk for diabetic CKD that reached end stage (requiring dialysis) than did non-obese adolescents.[9]

So what gives rise to the weight problems of our kids? Research and common sense tell us that our children eat poorly and sit too much. Here are some of the study results:

> **Kids get way too much salt.**
> The CDC determined that our little ones are eating as much salt as adults, with the average child taking in almost 3500 mg. per day—way over the 1500 mg. daily limit recommended for children. Some slug down over 8000 mg. of salt a day. They are stuffing themselves with processed meats (hotdogs, luncheon meat, bacon, pepperoni, sausage), fast food and restaurant items, snack foods, packaged and frozen meals. These are all loaded with salt.[10] Kids in the top quarter of salt consumption have double the risk of elevated blood pressure. Overweight and obese kids have 3½ times the risk.

Kids get way too much sugar.
Nearly 20 percent of a child's calories come from added sugars. About half of those sugar calories were swigged down in soft drinks. Shocking is that most of the added sugar calories were consumed in the home.[11] Even tots between ages 2 and 5 are given sugary drinks and are getting fat.[12]

Kids get too much screen time.
The presence of a TV or computer in a child's bedroom or otherwise easily accessible to the child is a significant risk factor for obesity and the diseases flowing from it. Kids watching TV or on computers spend less time on physical activity, eat fewer family meals, eat fewer vegetables, drink more sweetened beverages, snack more, and consume less healthy foods.[13]

Kids following DASH avoided weight gain.
Kids following a DASH-like diet (fruits, vegetables, whole grains) were compared with kids eating the customary SAD diet (fast foods, few fruits and vegetables, red meat, fatty food, salty stuff, and added sugars). The DASH group weighed less and were healthier.[14]

The bottom line: Stop with sweetened beverages. Kids love health-promoting smoothies, and you can't help but feel good about their increased consumption of wholesome fruits and vegetables. Make enough smoothie for two, so you can enjoy one with your child.

Part 2
Smoothies and Health

Improved health is in your control, and you begin here by enjoying the numerous kidney and heart benefits of regular consumption or fruits and vegetables. Plant-based foods provide ideal nutrition and have a detoxifying effect helpful in relieving disease states. These kidney-friendly smoothies are packed with antioxidants and phytonutrients that help protect you and your kidneys from degeneration and further disease.

Let's dig deeper into the make-up of kidney-healthy foods to see why fruits and vegetables are so magical.

CHAPTER 3:
EATS KIDNEYS LOVE

DASH for Health

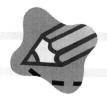

Most people with kidney disease can follow a normal—whoops, a healthful–diet without unusual restrictions, says the National Kidney Foundation.[1] A healthful diet is NOT the standard American diet (SAD), a diet crammed with greasy fast food; heavily laced with sodium and fat; loaded with processed and packaged concoctions; and then all washed down with sugary or artificially sweetened beverages. How can the body fight disease on such nutrient-devoid junk?

A diet that can improve kidney function is nutrient dense, filled with fruits and vegetables, nuts and seeds, whole grains, beans, low-fat dairy, and some fish. The NKF describes a healthful kidney diet for people in stages 1 through 4 of CKD to be the DASH diet.[2] The interesting thing about DASH is that it is great for anyone, not just kidney patients, and our smoothies are based on DASH principles.

DASH was born in the mid 1990's when a consortium of researchers from leading health organizations studied the effect of a diet rich in fruits, vegetables, nuts, beans, and seeds on blood pressure. The study was called **Dietary Approaches to Stop Hypertension (DASH)**.[3] After just eight weeks of eating the DASH diet, blood pressure levels among the study subjects fell.

Since that time, numerous other studies using DASH have confirmed its health effects, including studies showing that reducing sodium with DASH was even better at lowering blood pressure. DASH extends beyond blood pressure to help kidney disease, diabetes, obesity, kidney stones, gout, cardiovascular disease, cancer, and multiple other conditions.[4]

People (including kids) following a DASH diet have a lower incidence of CKD. For those already suffering from CKD, DASH can slow its progression and help lower proteinuria.[5]

> Researchers followed subjects ages 18 to 30 for 20 years. Subjects adhering most closely to the DASH diet were less likely to develop CKD and obesity. Subjects who had poor DASH adherence and were obese, smoked, or lacked exercise had a 337 percent increased risk for CKD.[6]

It's no wonder that leading health organizations heartily endorse DASH. The DASH diet is recommended by the NKF and the American Diabetes Association. It is approved by the National Heart, Lung and Blood Institute and the American Heart Association. DASH was highlighted in the 2010 Dietary Guidelines for Americans and also forms the basis for the USDA's My Plate.

DASH got a big plug when U.S. News & World Report rated it as "The Best Diet Overall" in 2014 and for several prior years. The rating was based on input from leading nutrition experts examining 32 popular diets. DASH quite simply is a great diet for good health.

DASH can accommodate late-stage CKD, too. Sure, some patients will need to limit potassium and phosphorus, but that leaves sufficient fruits and vegetables to help maintain health and strength. Talk with your renal dietitian about DASH and any modifications you need to make in view of your particular situation, and then select your smoothies from one (or more) of the three smoothie sections presented here.

By the way, the Mediterranean diet, a diet nearly identical to DASH, is also kidney protective. A recent study found that patients with Mediterranean-style eating habits (which would also be DASH-style eating habits) had a 50 percent reduced odds of developing CKD over the 7-year study, compared with patients not eating a diet high in fruits and vegetables and low in saturated fats. [7]

The primary difference between the DASH and Mediterranean diets is wine. Add a glass of wine a day to the DASH diet (in place of one fruit serving) and you have a Mediterranean diet.

For the full DASH diet, see Appendix A.

Renal Diet: A Confusing Label

Wait, you protest. Aren't I supposed to be on a renal diet? Kidney patients often say they follow a "renal diet," as if it were a single diet for all kidney patients. However, renal diets vary from stage to stage of CKD and are adjusted based on individual blood test results and type of kidney disease.

A renal diet in earlier stages of CKD is designed to preserve remaining kidney function and help reduce odds of cardiovascular events. So, a renal diet in stages 1-4 is the DASH diet for most patients, as recommended by the NKF.[1] In stage 5 of CKD, when dialysis is necessary, dietary restrictions are all about reducing death risk from heart disease caused by the kidneys' inability to control blood levels of certain chemicals, and a renal diet's components at that stage can change dramatically.

Nearly all kidney patients must reduce sodium intake, and this reduction is reflected in renal diets at any stage of CKD, including in the DASH diet. High blood pressure is destructive to both the kidneys and the cardiovascular system, and most kidney patients are plagued with it. But then, so are most American adults and a growing number of children, which is why we all should restrict sodium.

As kidneys deteriorate, they become unable to maintain proper balances of certain vital electrolytes in the body. Potassium and/or phosphorus levels can rise too high. Calcium can drop too low, as can vitamin D. So, a renal diet is adjusted to help compensate for these imbalances. The patient must limit intake of high potassium or high phosphorus foods, or must supplement with calcium or vitamin D.

The limiting of potassium (found in many delicious fruits and vegetables) and phosphorus (found primarily in dairy, meat and nuts) often signals to the kidney patient that life is truly changed by CKD. But, many wonderfully nutritious foods remain available.

In stage 5 and with dialysis, the renal diet becomes most challenging. Besides limitations on potassium and phosphorus, fluid intake is often restricted, depending on the type and frequency of dialysis chosen by the kidney patient. Salt needs may increase because of loss of sodium during dialysis sessions.

Continuing health in stage 5 is intimately tied to how well the dialysis patient adheres to the renal diet, and a renal dietitian is a must. The smoothies in the dialysis section of the book are dietitian approved and just might add variety to the dialysis patient's renal diet, as well as providing heart protection. Preserving good health is also vital to the dialysis patient's ability to qualify for and then receive a kidney for transplantation.

Antioxidants: Health Superheroes

Antioxidants are superheroes that counteract damaging oxidation constantly taking place in your body. During oxidation, harmful oxygen-containing molecules called **free radicals** form. Free radicals damage cells by altering their structure, their protein, and even their DNA.[1] The ultimate result? Disease—including kidney disease!

Some free radicals naturally form when cells metabolize food for energy or as an immune response to wipe out infectious bacteria and viruses. But, too many free radicals resulting from lousy food you've slogged down or exposure to environmental hazards such as tobacco smoke, radiation, and pollution set you up for multiple diseases and premature aging.

Why are free radicals so dangerous? In a nutshell, they are missing an electron, making them unstable. These restless molecules then act like thieves, stealing electrons from other molecules, turning them into new free radicals. The new free radicals then steal from other molecules, again making new free radicals, and so on.

Too many free radicals are trouble, and your body utilizes antioxidants to control them. Your cells make some antioxidants but rely on wholesome plant foods for others. The antioxidant superheroes seek out excess free radicals, neutralizing them so they can do no more damage. If free radicals accumulate faster than the body can mop them up (think colas, hot dogs, and similar crap food), dangerous **oxidative stress** occurs.

Oxidative stress contributes to various chronic diseases and conditions, including kidney disease, heart disease, diabetes, cancer, aging, Alzheimer's.[2] Several studies tie oxidative stress to kidney disease and development of cardiovascular disease.[3] So, oxidative stress-fighting antioxidants are particularly important to kidney patients.

Thousands of different antioxidants exist in fruits, vegetables, and whole grains, as well as in coffee, tea, and wine. Antioxidants have assigned jobs. Some suppress formation of free radicals, while others destroy free radicals before they can do damage, or work to repair damage once it is done. When we load up on antioxidant-rich plants, we're shielded against free radicals that can inflame our artery linings, damage our kidneys' glomeruli, and increase our odds of becoming obese and diabetic.

> Think of antioxidants as Viagra® for kidneys. Up your intake to enjoy a "rise" in kidney function.

Some familiar nutrients that act as antioxidants are vitamins C and E, beta carotene, and selenium. Numerous others are **phytochemicals** from plants, and still others are enzymes. Junk foods contain little or no antioxidants and even contribute to formation of free radicals.

Getting more antioxidants is great for health so long as the antioxidants come from real food. Popping an antioxidant pill to get a high dose of a particular antioxidant can have adverse effects (high-dose beta-carotene can increase cancer risk, for example).[4] Antioxidants work with the numerous other components existing in whole foods to deliver their disease-fighting impact.

Phytochemicals: Keys to Better Health

Phytochemicals, also called phytonutrients, are chemicals found in plants ("phyto" is derived from the Greek word for plant) and protect the plants by helping them fight disease. They do the same for us when we consume the plants.

Phytochemicals give fruits and vegetables their vibrant colors. More than 8,000 phytochemicals are identified to date, and many are antioxidants. The deeper the plant color, the greater the phytochemical/antioxidant content. A single serving of vegetables may contain over 100 different phytochemicals that can shield us from those dangerous free radicals. So, eat your colors: and no, we are not talking about M&M's®! Think: dark green lettuces, luscious red fruit, deep blue blueberries....

Some phytochemicals you may recognize are:

Carotenoids
Found in carrots, cantaloupe, sweet potatoes, and fall squash, and may protect against kidney disease and cardiovascular disease.

Glucosinolates
Found in vegetables, and may help the liver in detoxification. They help regulate white blood cells involved in immunity, and may help reduce tumor growth.

Limonoids
Found in the peel of citrus fruits, these phytochemicals appear to protect lung tissue.

Lycopene
Found in tomatoes and watermelon, and may protect against cancer.

> **Phenols and polyphenols**
> Found in green tea, these protect plants from chemical damage and may do the same in humans. Phenols are thought to protect against cancer.

The evidence is that people who consume a diet rich in plant foods (fruits, vegetables, whole grains, nuts/seeds) have lower incidence of many disorders, including kidney disease, urinary tract infections, kidney stones, high blood pressure, obesity, heart disease, and cancer.[1] Folks eating lots of produce also tend to live longer, healthier lives.[2] So, eat up—or, in the case of smoothies, drink up!

Fiber: Disease Fighter

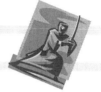

Fruits and vegetables are great sources of fiber, and packing your diet with fiber-rich foods could improve health and kidney status. A high fiber diet is associated with a decreased risk of CKD.[1] In individuals with CKD, consuming high fiber foods seems to lessen destructive internal inflammation and all-cause mortality.[2] In sad contrast, low-fiber diets up the risk for kidney disease.[3]

Fiber also lowers risk of death from cardiovascular disease, including high blood pressure, clogged arteries, and heart attacks, all so common in kidney patients. Fiber helps to lower cholesterol levels, control blood-sugar levels, and maintain a healthy digestive tract. Fiber consumption also assists in reducing a number of chronic diseases that plague kidney patients, such as obesity, type 2 diabetes, and several cancers.

The two types of fiber are **soluble** and **insoluble.** Soluble fiber absorbs water, thereby aiding to slow absorption of glucose. Slowing the rate of glucose absorption from the intestines is a good thing. This gives the liver a chance to metabolize what is coming in, so excess glucose doesn't flood the bloodstream and trigger an over-release of insulin.

Soluble fiber's ability to lower cholesterol and blood pressure is beneficial to kidneys and the heart. Stroke risk is lower in fiber eaters.[4]

Insoluble fiber does not dissolve in water and is not even digested. Because it is not digested, insoluble fiber has a bulking, laxative effect that speeds passage of food and waste through your gut for great bowel movements and reduced risk of cancer. Both types of fiber are an unbeatable pair that work together for good health, including kidney health.

Soluble Fiber (Absorbs water)	Insoluble Fiber (Doesn't absorb water)
apples, beans, blueberries, carrots, cucumbers, dried peas, flaxseeds, lentils, nuts, oat bran, oat cereal, oatmeal, oranges, pears, psyllium, strawberries	barley, broccoli, brown rice, bulgar, cabbage, carrots, celery, corn bran, couscous, cucumbers, dark leafy vegetables, fruit, green beans, nuts, onions, root vegetables, tomatoes, wheat bran, whole grains, whole wheat, zucchini

The U.S. Department of Agriculture's 2010 Dietary Guidelines for Americans recommend 25 to 38 grams of fiber per day.[5] Sadly, only five percent of Americans meet that goal. The average intake in the U.S. is only about 15 grams per day.

Why do we fall woefully short on this beneficial nutrient? It's simple, but two parts. First, we've substituted processed foods for the real stuff. Food manufacturing strips bran from our whole grains to create half-foods for a longer shelf life. When the bran is removed, the product you eat doesn't linger in your intestines but hits your bloodstream quickly. That means higher insulin peaks and increased diabetes and obesity risks.

Food Item	Grams/Fiber
Apple (1 small)	4
Raspberries (1 cup)	9
Blackberries (1 cup)	7
Avocado (1/2)	5
Pear (1 small)	5
Black beans (1/2 cup)	8
Kidney beans (1/2 cup)	7
Ground flaxseed (3 T.)	8
Almonds (23)	4
Sweet potato, w/skin (1 small)	4
Broccoli (2 spears)	3

A second reason we are not getting our fiber is that we simply don't eat our plant foods. The richest sources of fiber are fruits, vegetables, whole grains, nuts, and legumes (beans). Sure, a renal diet can interfere with the inability of late-stage kidney patients to enjoy many potassium-rich plant foods, but that still leaves lots of lower-potassium plant choices that are loaded with fiber.

Kidney-friendly smoothies are the perfect solution to getting enough fiber in your diet—and you'll enjoy drinking them! Each smoothie is made with fiber-rich produce, and each recipe includes the grams of fiber so you can add your smoothie fiber amount to the fiber count in other foods you eat during the day to reach the daily fiber goal of 25 to 38 grams.

Chapter 4: Slowing Kidney Damage with Produce

Acidosis: Internal Burn

People with kidney disease often have **metabolic acidosis**, a condition in which their blood is slightly acidic rather than alkaline. Acidosis contributes to internal inflammation, leaching of calcium from bone, and raising the likelihood of other disease conditions, including diabetes, high blood pressure, and heart disease—the very ailments so common in kidney patients.

You've probably heard of the pH (power of hydrogen) scale, which is a scale used to measure the acidity or alkalinity of substances. The **pH scale** ranges from 0-14. A substance with a pH of 0-7 is considered acidic. A pH above 7 is alkaline or base. Distilled water has a pH of exactly 7 and is considered neutral. Serum pH that is slightly alkaline (7.35-7.45) is normal in people with well-functioning kidneys, and that slightly alkaline pH is best for wellness.

Kidneys are responsible for maintaining a proper acid/base equilibrium and are great at the job when functioning properly. If our diets are more acid-producing, healthy kidneys filter out the excess acid into urine. As kidney function deteriorates, kidneys become unable to filter excess acid, leading to undesirable acidosis.

> Battery acid is a 1 on the pH scale. Cola is almost as acidic, at a 2.5 pH.

Drugs we take and our diets impact our internal acid/base balance. When metabolized, these items break down into residues that register acid or base. Alkaline-inducing foods such as vegetables and fruits decrease dietary acid load and can help slow kidney disease.[1]

Unfortunately, the "standard American diet" (SAD) imposes a tremendous acid load on the body. Acid-forming foods include meat, dairy, sugar of any sort, processed foods, soft drinks, and caffeinated beverages. Such foods strain damaged kidneys that are already struggling to balance pH blood levels.

The result of acidic-food overload is an acidic internal environment, rather than acidic urine. Acidosis from a poor diet accelerates progression of kidney disease and increases the kidney patient's susceptibility to other diseases.[2]

> In a study of 249 CKD patients, high dietary acid levels were linked with accelerated kidney function decline. Patients with elevated acid levels had an increased risk of CKD progression compared to patients with low acid levels. [3]

The NKF says that in kidney disease, acidosis is associated with "bone disease, muscle wasting, chronic inflammation, impaired glucose homeostasis, impaired cardiac function, progression of CKD, and increased mortality." [4] Whew!

Kidney patients are often prescribed sodium bicarbonate (baking soda) tablets to counteract acidosis prevalent in kidney disease. This alkaline substance neutralizes or balances acid. However, kidney patients often cannot tolerate the sodium load from the pills. Developing research indicates that consuming fruits and vegetables works just as well as bicarbonate pills in reducing acid overload.[5] Moreover, fruits and vegetables supply vital nutrients not available in a baking soda pill and taste a whole lot better.

> To test whether fruits and vegetables protect kidney health, researchers had 23 hypertensive patients consume extra fruits and vegetables, 23 patients received oral alkaline drugs, and 25 patients received nothing. One year later, kidney disease progressed in the group receiving nothing, but kidney health was preserved in the fruit/vegetable and the oral drug groups.[6]

A recent study found that nearly one-third of kidney **transplant recipients** exhibits acidosis. Acidosis may contribute to loss of the transplanted organ. Recipients who modified their diets to increase fruits and vegetables and decrease animal protein improved acid-base balances.[7]

The bottom line: Eating a predominantly alkaline diet of plant-based foods improves metabolic acidosis and can provide kidney protection. Substitute healthful, produce-filled smoothies for SAD meals to help your kidneys win the pH battle, thereby extending the life of your kidneys and increasing your overall odds for better health.

Alkaline-Forming Foods*

Fruit: Most fruits are alkaline-inducing and loaded with antioxidants, fiber, and valuable nutrients, so choose a variety. While some fruits are mildly acidic-inducing, their nutrient content weighs in favor of consuming them. (Stay away from starfruit, which is toxic to kidneys).

Grains: Grains are important for their phytochemicals and fiber, and most are alkaline inducing. Some (wheat, oats, brown rice) are mildly acidic-inducing but remain valuable diet additions.

Lemons, limes: These are listed separately from fruits because they are little alkaline-inducing powerhouses. They are foolers because they are acidic but have an alkaline effect when ingested. Try the juice (and zest) of a lime in a glass of warm water every morning for a refreshing start to the day.

Nuts, seeds: Nuts and seeds contain powerful antioxidants and heart-healthy oils. Most are alkaline inducing. Those that are mildly acid-producing are still valuable components to an overall healthy diet.

Oils: Try extra virgin olive oil and nut oils.

Vegetables: Nearly all vegetables are alkaline inducing so enjoy a variety. Choose dark green lettuces (particularly kale, collards, cabbage, spinach, mustard greens); bright orange sweet potatoes and carrots; deep red, yellow, and green peppers. Consume a variety daily.

*May be consumed freely, except in late-stage CKD

Acid-Forming Foods**

Animal protein: Meat (all kinds), dairy (cheese is highly acid inducing). While fish is mildly acid-inducing, it has health attributes that make it an occasional good choice.

Chemicals: Drugs, tobacco, pesticides, pollution, preservatives, MSG.

Condiments: Ketchup, mustard, mayonnaise, margarine, refined vegetable oils.

Processed products: If it doesn't look the way it did when it was harvested, it's probably processed.

Refined grains: White flour, white bread, white rice, packaged foods containing processed grains.

Sugar: All kinds, including honey, corn syrup, molasses, sugar substitutes, any sugar in drinks or packaged products.

Sweet drinks: Sodas, colas, sweetened drinks, punch juice, fruit juice (even 100percent fruit).

**Consume only in moderation, or eliminate

Inflammation: Internal Attack

Chronic inflammation is implicated in a long list of diseases and disorders, including CKD, diabetes, heart disease, high blood pressure, metabolic syndrome, cancer, and on and on. We're not talking about the throbbing, red, swollen inflammation you experience after a paper cut or ankle sprain. Such acute inflammation is short-lived and localized, lasting only until the injury heals.

Chronic inflammation is a long-term, internal attack on your body's cells. Over time, the inflammatory attack may result in disease. The disease then aggravates inflammation, worsening health and furthering aggravating inflammation. Ah, a vicious cycle.

Even in its early stages, CKD is a persistent inflammatory state.[1] As CKD progresses, both inflammation and oxidative stress increase. Health plummets further as a result.

Inflammation is often measured by determining the level of **C-reactive protein** in the blood (serum CRP). Elevated serum CRP is an indication of inflammation and a strong predictor of risk for cardiovascular events (heart attack, stroke) and early death in kidney patients.[2] Lowering serum CRP in CKD is linked to reduced inflammation and decreased risk of early mortality.[3] Likewise, lowering inflammation in kidney disease appears to preserve kidney function.[4]

One way to lower inflammation in kidney disease is to increase consumption of dietary fiber.[5] Fiber is abundant in vegetables, fruits, whole grains, nuts, seeds, beans—and kidney-friendly smoothies.

Another way to reduce inflammation is by losing weight. Fat cells spew inflammation-causing markers into the bloodstream. Besides kidney disease, these markers can lead to insulin resistance and diabetes.[6]

Switching to a produce-based diet is a great way to control inflammation and weight. The smoothies suggested here also give you a vital extra bump in fiber.

Uric Acid: Contributes to Acidosis

Kidney patients commonly have high **uric acid** levels **(hyperuricemia)**, which seem to accelerate loss of kidney function.[1] Hyperuricemia is also common in patients after kidney transplantation and plays a strong role in gout, kidney stones, and heart disease. A serum uric acid level of 6 mg/dL is the goal.[2] Have yours measured.

Uric acid is a byproduct of the breakdown of purines, a chemical normally found in body cells and in certain foods. Purines are important because they help form our DNA, as well as having other vital functions. The uric acid by-product, though, is toxic.

Working kidneys are able to eliminate the majority of the uric acid created from the body's use of purines. Once again, though, as kidney function deteriorates, kidneys lose that ability, and uric acid levels build in the blood. Uric acid obviously is acidic, increasing internal inflammation, acidosis, and disease risk.

Lowering serum uric acid levels seems to slow progression of kidney disease and proteinuria, as well as reduce risk of cardiovascular disease.[3]

> In a study of 16,186 patients, those who achieved a serum uric acid of less than 6 mg/dL demonstrated a 37% reduction in progression of kidney disease.[4]

Limiting foods with high amounts of purines lowers uric acid levels. Purines are found in high concentration in meats. Uric acid levels and risk of CKD are also higher in people who consume sugar and both sweetened and diet beverages.[5]

Generally, plant-based foods are low in purines (although, moderate amounts of purines are found in some, such as spinach, mushrooms, beans, wheat). So, it's not surprising that fruits and vegetable consumption is tied to lower uric acid levels.[6]

Eating more fruits and vegetables and limiting meat and sugar consumption are sound strategies to slow CKD progression and acidosis by lessening uric acid levels. Think of this as you drink a delicious, produce-based smoothie.

Be Protein Picky

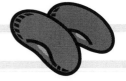

Myths abound when it comes to **protein**. Many believe that meat is the only good source of protein, and the more eaten the better. That is poor thinking when it comes to kidney health. Plant foods provide plenty of high quality protein that is much kinder to your kidneys. Perhaps, that is why vegetarians who don't eat meat have lower rates of CKD and live longer than meat eaters.[1]

The National Kidney Foundation recommends that individuals with CKD—even in the earliest stages—limit protein consumption to less than "0.8 g/kg body weight per day."[2] That translates into

55 grams of total protein per day for a 150-pound person. The 0.8g/kg limit is the same limit recommended by the Institute of Medicine for healthy adult.[3] So, kidney patients shouldn't feel slighted.

If CKD is progressive (GFR worsens over time) or if you have advanced CKD and are not on dialysis, the NKF recommends limiting daily protein to 0.6 g/kg of body weight.[4] That is 41 grams of total protein per day for a 150-pound person.

To put this in perspective, that 16-ounce t-bone from your favorite steak house can contain 122 grams of protein (2 to 3 days worth of protein). A roasted chicken breast has about 29 grams; an 8-ounce glass of milk gives you 8 grams; and, a slice of whole wheat bread contains 4 grams of protein. Even a serving of orange juice provides 2 protein grams.[5]

Most kidney patients unwittingly eat twice the recommended amount of protein per day, even in CKD stages 3 and 4.[6] Thus, counting protein grams in the daily diet makes sense.

Research is clear that too much protein, particularly meat protein, in the diet of a person with CKD stresses kidneys. Protein contains nitrogen, which is converted in the body to waste products such as **urea** and ammonia. These substances are toxic, and healthy kidneys can filter them from the blood into urine.

Poorly-functioning kidneys have lost the necessary number of filtering units (glomeruli) to fully excrete the nitrogen wastes, allowing them to accumulate in the body. As a result, the kidney patient may suffer loss of appetite, fatigue, headaches, nausea, increasing proteinuria, and further kidney damage. When CKD hits stage 5, uremic poisoning can result from the build-up of urea. A function of dialysis is to remove nitrogen-based toxins.

Failing to consume sufficient protein is just as dangerous as having too much. Too little protein leads to muscle loss and malnutrition, which is common in later-stage kidney patients and is a powerful predictor of increased risk for further disease and early death.[7] Protein is required for survival. It is utilized for repair of body tissues, cell growth, wound healing, and fighting infections. Some kidney conditions, such as nephrotic syndrome, result in lose of large amounts of protein in urine, leaving an even greater need for the nutrient.

A powerful way to obtain necessary protein while protecting kidneys is to use fruits, vegetables, grains, and nuts/seeds as protein sources rather than meat. Besides being acid-inducing, animal protein seems to increase progression of CKD. In contrast, alkaline-inducing produce as the protein source results in decreased kidney injury and improvement in metabolic acidosis.[8]

The newest research supports consuming produce rather than meat for protein to increase survival in kidney disease.

> Researchers looked at diets of over 1,100 kidney patients. For each 10-gram rise in consumption of vegetable protein (rather than animal protein) per day, patients had a 14% lowered risk of dying during the study.[9]

Relying on produce rather than meat for protein might decrease uremic toxins, kidney damage, and CKD progression.[10]

Some authors suggest that if people with very advanced CKD severely limit protein intake, they might delay dialysis for a few months.[11] The NKF doesn't support that hypothesis. Most research on severe protein restriction involved animals or very small numbers of people. Certainly, protein restriction of less than the NKF's recommended 0.8 g/kg and 0.6 g/kg requires careful monitoring by a nephrologist and renal dietitian.

The kidney-protective smoothies here utilize plant protein and low-fat dairy. The recipes for dialysis patients will include higher plant protein amounts because of the greater potential for malnutrition and muscle wasting in dialysis as compared to earlier CKD stages.

Those Pesky Electrolytes

Electrolytes are minerals (such as sodium, potassium, phosphorus, calcium) vital for most actions involved in living, including heartbeat, nerve cell actions, brain function, and muscle movement. We obtain these chemicals from our diet, and we must maintain a proper internal balance for good health.

Kidneys are responsible for maintaining that proper balance by filtering into urine excess electrolytes accumulating in the blood. Too much of any one electrolyte becomes toxic. As CKD advances, damaged kidneys lose that filtering ability. So, late-stage kidney patients often must reduce their intake of certain foods to keep electrolyte levels in normal ranges.

Sodium—Shake the Kidney-Damaging Habit

It is no surprise that both the NKF and the American Heart Association come down hard on our salt habit. Most health organizations agree that kidney patients (as well as anyone over age 50, African-Americans, and people with hypertension or diabetes) should limit sodium intake to a maximum of 1500 mg. per day.[1] That applies to 70 percent of us. Yet, most Americans consume a startling 3500 mg. each day, well over double the recommended limit.[2]

We actually need only 500 mg. of daily sodium, and we get that amount naturally from wholesome food. Consuming processed, packaged items, fast food, and restaurant fare propels our sodium intake into the danger zone. Persistently high sodium levels in blood can lead to edema, higher blood pressure, heart failure, difficulty breathing, and even death.

Limiting sodium is particularly important in kidney disease, in part because most kidney patients have high blood pressure. Cutting sodium lowers pressure.[3] Sodium may directly impair kidney function and leaches calcium from bones. Reducing sodium lowers proteinuria and slows kidney damage.[4]

The newest research emphasizes the power of salt reduction in prolonging the lives of kidney patients, lowering blood pressure, and substantially decreasing proteinuria.

A study cited by the NKF in its newest CKD guidelines found that a "salt-restricted diet significantly reduced 24-hour urinary protein ...by 19 percent and led to a fall in systolic blood pressure of 8 mm Hg."[5]

In the Low SALT CKD study, 20 patients were put on a high-salt diet (up to 4600 mg/day) for 2 weeks and then put on a low-salt diet (below 1500 mg/day) for 2 weeks. The low-salt diet lowered blood pressure by 10/4 mm Hg. and cut proteinuria by 50 percent. Maintaining the low-salt diet could reduce risk of ESRD and early death by 30 percent.[6]

As emphasized previously, following a DASH diet with lowered sodium intake is shown to improve hypertension and albumin/creatinine ratios. It's the produce in our DASH-inspired smoothies that drives these beneficial effects--the antioxidants, phytochemicals, potassium, magnesium, and fiber in fruits and vegetables.

People with CKD are often salt-sensitive, making salt restriction even more important.

Potassium Power!

Potassium is critical for good health, and so long as your kidneys function moderately, you can heartily enjoy potassium-rich foods. Potassium aids in maintaining blood pressure by counteracting the negative effect of too much sodium.[7] It is involved in proper nerve, cell, muscle, and bone function, as well as fluid balance.

Despite the importance of potassium in these vital functions, Americans eat less than half the recommended 4700 milligrams per day. Potassium is commonly found in fruits and vegetables. The USDA's 2010 Dietary Guidelines recommend at least seven servings of fruits and vegetables each day to meet our potassium needs. The average American consumes less than four servings, and that's counting French fries and ketchup.[8]

Most kidney patients can enjoy as many potassium-rich foods as they want without any known danger from excess potassium. Even ailing kidneys maintain the ability to excrete excess potassium for some time, allowing blood levels to stay in the proper 3.5 to 5.2 mEq/L range.

However, as kidney disease advances to end-stage, the ability to filter excess potassium decreases, causing **hyperkalemia** (excess potassium in blood). Also, certain kidney diseases and some medications may raise potassium levels. Hyperkalemia is dangerous and can cause irregular heartbeats, heart failure, and death.

Dialysis patients who have little or no remaining kidney function must closely monitor potassium consumption to avoid hyperkalemia. At no point, though, will you need to avoid all plant sources of this valuable mineral.

The NKF's guidelines encourage consumption of vegetables and fruits and the DASH diet for kidney patients in stages 1-4 of CKD.[9] It is only when blood tests indicate blood potassium levels are too high that diet must be modified to prevent hyperkalemia. So long as you are not to that point, enjoy potassium-loaded produce. Your motto could be "less salt, more potassium."

Potassium-Rich Foods[10]
(greater than 200 milligrams per portion)

The following table lists foods that are high in potassium. The portion size is ½ cup unless otherwise stated. **Please be sure to check portion sizes.** While all foods on this list are high in potassium, some are higher than others.

Fruits	Vegetables	Other
Apricot, raw (2 md)	Acorn Squash	Bran/Bran products
dried (5 halves)	Artichoke	Chocolate (1½-2 oz.)
Avocado (¼)	Bamboo Shoots	Granola
Banana (½)	Baked Beans	Milk, all types (1 c.)
Cantaloupe	Butternut Squash	Molasses (1 T.)
Dates (5)	Refried Beans	Nuts, Seeds (1 oz.)
Dried fruits	Beets, fresh then boiled	Peanut Butter (2 T.)
Figs, dried	Black Beans	Salt Substitutes/ Lite Salt
Grapefruit Juice	Broccoli, cooked	Salt Free Broth
Honeydew	Brussels Sprouts	Yogurt
Kiwi (1 med.)	Chinese Cabbage	Snuff/ Chewing Tobacco
Mango (1 med.)	Carrots, raw	Nutritional Supplements (Use only under the direction of your doctor or dietitian)
Nectarine (1 med.)	Dried Beans and Peas	
Orange (1 med.)	Greens, except Kale	
Orange Juice	Hubbard Squash	
Papaya (½)	Kohlrabi	
Pomegranate (1)	Lentils	
Pomegranate Juice	Legumes	
Prunes	White Mushrooms, cooked	
Prune Juice	Okra	
Raisins	Parsnips	
	Potatoes, white and sweet	
	Pumpkin	
	Rutabagas	
	Spinach, cooked	
	Tomatoes/Tomato products	
	Vegetable Juices	

Low-Potassium Foods[10]

The following table list foods which are low in potassium.
A portion is ½ cup unless otherwise noted. **Eating more than 1 portion can make a lower potassium food into a higher potassium food.**

Fruits	Vegetables	Other
Apple (1 med.)	Alfalfa sprouts	Rice
Apple Juice	Asparagus (6 spears)	Noodles
Applesauce	Beans, green or wax	Pasta
Apricots, canned in juice	Cabbage, green and red	Bread and bread products (not whole grains)
Blackberries	Carrots, cooked	
Blueberries	Cauliflower	
Cherries	Celery (1 stalk)	Cake: angel, yellow
Cranberries	Corn, fresh (½ ear) frozen	
Fruit Cocktail		Coffee: **limit to 8 ounces**
Grapes	Cucumber	
Grape Juice	Eggplant	Pies without chocolate or high potassium fruit
Grapefruit (½)	Kale	
Mandarin Oranges	Lettuce	
Peaches, fresh (1 sml.) canned (½ c.)	Mixed Vegetables	
	White Mushrooms, raw	Cookies without nuts or chocolate
Pears, fresh (1 sml.) canned (½ c.)	Onions	
	Parsley	Tea: **limit to 16 ounces**
Pineapple	Peas, green	
Pineapple Juice	Peppers	
Plums (1)	Radish	
Raspberries	Rhubarb	
Strawberries	Water Chestnuts, canned	
Tangerine (1)	Watercress	
Watermelon (**limit to 1 cup**)	Yellow Squash	
	Zucchini Squash	

Phosphorus, Calcium's Partner

Phosphorus is the second most abundant mineral in the body, right behind calcium. About 85 percent of phosphorus is in bones and teeth, where it works with calcium. Phosphorus also helps form cell membranes, assists to store energy, aids in neutralizing too-acidic blood, and is part of your DNA.

Adults need 700 mg. of phosphorus daily, but on average Americans get about twice that amount. As with all electrolytes, phosphates must exist in the blood at a precise level. Kidneys maintain that delicate balance by excreting excess phosphates into urine.

When poorly-functioning kidneys fail to maintain phosphorus balance, the mineral can accumulate in the blood. A normal phosphorus blood level is 3.5 to 5.5 mg/dL. Consistently high phosphorus levels accelerate loss of calcium from bones, which can deposit in the blood vessels and heart. You know what that means—increased risk of osteoporosis, heart attack, and stroke.

> *Phosphates added to soft drinks, processed meats, cheese and baked goods increase odds of faster-than-normal decline in kidney function.*[13]

Excess phosphorus raises risk of CKD and heart attacks in otherwise healthy individuals, and accelerates progression of kidney disease in those who already have it.[11] Meat and dairy are primary sources of phosphorus, as are certain beans and nuts.

Eating processed foods, including fast food, prepared frozen foods, and packaged meats, is also a phosphorus problem.[12] These foods nearly always contain phosphate additives, causing kidney and heart mischief. The NKF recommends limiting these foods early in CKD to help preserve kidney function. Packaged, processed foods generally aren't good for us anyway.

Kidney patients who obtain their phosphorus from vegetables rather than from meat and processed foods sustain proper blood levels longer into kidney disease.[13] However, late-stage kidney patients with little or no kidney function often must limit phosphorus-containing foods and might also take phosphate binders to reduce phosphate levels.

Nearly all fruits and vegetables are low in phosphorus. The only exception are beans, nuts/seeds, bran, and whole wheat. The highest phosphorus-containing foods are animal products—yep, meat and cheese. Processed and packaged products and colas are high in phosphorus because it is added in several forms as a preservative.

The National Kidney Foundation provides this listing of high phosphorus foods that late-stage kidney patients may need to limit, depending on blood levels of phosphorus.[14]

High Phosphorus Foods to Limit or Avoid[15]

Beverages	Ale, beer, chocolate drinks, cocoa, drinks made with milk, dark colas, canned iced teas
Dairy Products	Cheese, cottage cheese, custard, ice cream, milk, pudding, cream soups, yogurt
Protein	Carp, crayfish, beef liver, chicken liver, fish roe, organ meats, oysters, sardines
Vegetables	Dried beans and peas, baked beans, black beans, chick peas, garbanzo beans, kidney beans, lentils, limas, northern beans, pork 'n' beans, split peas, soybeans
Other foods	Bran cereals, brewer's yeast, caramels, nuts, seeds, wheat germ, whole grain products

Calcium

Calcium, the most abundant mineral in the body, is located primarily in bones and teeth. Calcium works with phosphorus to provide strength and structure to bones and teeth. About one percent of your calcium is located in your blood, muscles, and tissues to assist with blood vessel contraction, blood clotting, and nervous system transmittal.

We obtain valuable calcium from our diets. Milk, yogurt, and cheese are main sources of calcium, but dark green vegetables also supply some. Unfortunately for kidney patients, consuming calcium isn't enough if the calcium is not absorbed by the body, which it isn't without the help of the active form of vitamin D.

Recall that in kidney disease, ailing kidneys lose the ability to manufacture **calcitriol** (the active version of vitamin D). Calcitriol normally stimulates your intestines to absorb calcium and phosphorus from diet to maintain healthy levels in blood and bones. Without adequate calcitriol, calcium blood levels become erratic.

To compensate, calcium is leached from bones to raise blood levels. This leaching can lead to brittle and weak bones. Moreover, the leached calcium in the blood gets deposited into blood vessels and the heart, increasing risk for cardiovascular disease. To help prevent this leaching, your nephrologist may prescribe a calcitriol analogue to compensate for the hormone your body can no longer make in sufficient quantities.

Each kidney-friendly smoothie recipe includes the amount of nutrients so you can keep track of intake. No smoothie contains excessive sodium, because fruits and vegetables are naturally low in sodium.

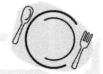

Food After a Kidney Transplant

Most kidney patients are thrilled to receive a donated kidney. Life after kidney transplantation is almost normal, unlike life on dialysis. Diet goes back to normal, too, a wonderful treat to long-suffering kidney patients. However, "back to normal" may be a mistake if "normal" is the SAD (standard American diet) way of eating that may have led to CKD in the first place.

Following my transplant surgery, the surgeon told me I could now "eat whatever I wanted." I actually had eaten my normal, largely vegetarian diet prior to surgery and never needed to alter my diet because of CKD. Blood levels of potassium and phosphorus stayed in proper ranges even when I entered CKD stage 5. In any event, the advice of my totally handsome surgeon was not good when you consider the diabetes, obesity, and hypertension epidemics driven largely by the standard American diet.

Healthful dietary choices by kidney transplant recipients are critical for the health of both the transplanted kidney (graft) and the recipient. Because transplantation is only a treatment and not a cure, the recipient still has CKD with its associated risks. The immunosuppressant drugs we must take can increase likelihood of certain health complications. Fortunately, a diet high in produce goes far to counter potential health complications. Common post-transplant complications include:

Acidosis

Over 30 percent of transplant recipients have acidosis. Recall that acidosis is a disturbance of the blood acid-base balance and is linked to a diet high in acid-inducing foods, such as cheese and meat, and low in alkaline-inducing fruits and vegetables. Acidosis increases risk of proteinuria and progression of CKD pre-transplant and post-transplant. It also can raise odds of graft failure.[1] Increasing fruits and vegetables and limiting consumption of animal protein seem to improve acidosis in transplant recipients.[2]

Cardiovascular Disease

Cardiovascular disease remains a serious threat after transplantation. It causes the of death about one-third of recipients.[3] Factors like proteinuria, hypertension, high lipid levels, and diabetes are all tied to risk of heart and vessel issues.

Nearly all transplant recipients have high cholesterol, which can be aggravated by immunosuppressants, as well as poor diet, diabetes, and obesity. The NKF recommends a DASH-like diet high in produce to lower cholesterol.[4]

A good diet of fruits, vegetables, nuts, fiber works to lower all cardiovascular risk factors after transplant surgery, including hypertension. About 80 percent of transplant recipients have hypertension, and it is associated with increased risk of graft failure.[5]

NODAT

New onset diabetes after transplantation (NODAT) also increases likelihood of cardiovascular events, loss of graft, and early death. NODAT is estimated to occur soon after transplantation. At 36 months following transplant, over 40 percent of recipients have NODAT.[6] Immunosuppressant drugs (particularly, tacrolimus and prednisone) can increase risk of NODAT, making a healthful diet even more important.

Weight Gain

About half of transplant recipients gain weight after surgery. The average weight gain is 10 percent of body weight the first year. Some of this relates to steroid immunosuppression, which is being used less often, thank goodness. Weight gain is also driven by the renewed appetite recipients enjoy. Watching weight obviously is critical to avoid obesity, diabetes, cardiovascular disease, and injury to the graft.

Bone Loss

Bone loss is common in kidney disease, carrying through post-transplant. Some immunosuppressants seem to contribute to bone loss. A diet with adequate calcium, phosphorus, and vitamin D is used to help relieve the issue.

Vitamin D deficiency appears in most kidney patients at the time of transplantation. Most Americans are vitamin D deficient if you listen to many experts. Recent research suggests vitamin D deficiency may result in damage to the graft and a lower GFR one year after transplantation, not something recipients want.[7]

Vitamin D Sources

- ✓ Sunlight
- ✓ Fatty fish
- ✓ Seafood
- ✓ Fortified milk products
- ✓ Avocados
- ✓ Broccoli
- ✓ Carrots
- ✓ Mushrooms
- ✓ Eggs

Have your vitamin D level checked and work with your doctor to raise it, if necessary. Focus on consuming vitamin D rich foods, too.

Infections/Cancer

Infections will kill 21 percent of recipients, and cancer another 10 percent.[8] Risk of infections and cancer are increased by the immunosuppressants. However, practicing appropriate safeguards (don't smoke, watch sun exposure, avoid crowds), including healthy eating, is protection against both.

Chapter 5:
Top Kidney-Protection Tips

Not on dialysis? Then you might slow the progression of kidney disease. Here are the top 10 habits of people who know how to guard kidney health–habits you can develop.

Tip 1 — Feast on Vegetables and Fruits

A DASH-like eating plan, loaded with vegetables and fruits, is a kidney's best friend. The standard American diet increases the likelihood of developing kidney disease and then having it worsen.

Fruits and vegetables help neutralize acidosis, a disease-aggravating internal state. They counteract internal inflammation and can help lower proteinuria, blood pressure, and obesity and diabetes risks. The numerous antioxidants, phytochemicals, enzymes, and related nutrients in fruits and vegetables are a fountain of longevity and the best protection we have against multiple disease conditions.

Tip 2 — Drink Water

Yep, slug down clean, plain water, and lots of it. Early research ties drinking water to lowered risk of CKD. In the studies, drinking 4 or slightly more liters of water each day offered the best kidney protection. Consuming this much water, of course, is not possible for dialysis patients or others with liquid restrictions. So, check with your doctor before changing your water habits. At a minimum, replace sodas and sweetened beverages with water. Your overall health and kidney function will reflect the improvement.

Tip 3 — Lower Blood Pressure

High blood pressure is a rapid kidney killer. Ignoring it for even a short time allows it to destroy delicate glomeruli in kidneys, reducing kidney function. A major contributor to raised blood pressure is sodium. Nearly all the salt we consume is metabolized by the kidneys. Excess salt intake makes kidneys work harder and can lead to kidney damage and increased blood pressure. Reduce total sodium intake to no more than 1500 mg a day, unless your doctor instructs otherwise.

Also, monitor your pressure twice daily in the peace and quiet of your home. Call your doctor if readings stay up over a few days. Take all antihypertensive meds as prescribed, and get your produce. Fruits and vegetables are repeatedly shown to lower blood pressure. Also, relax and enjoy a good night's sleep—every night.

Tip 4 — Reduce Proteinuria

You just may have some power over the quantity of protein spilled by your kidneys. Proteinuria is never good. Even a little proteinuria raises cardiovascular risk. The greater the proteinuria, the worse the CKD outcome. Likewise, reducing proteinuria slows CKD progression, and diet can help. Diets high in fruits and vegetables are linked to decreased protein in urine.

Tip 5 — Cut Protein

Protein, particularly from red and processed meats, is stressful to damaged kidneys. Digestion of meat and use by your cells creates nitrogen-containing wastes that faulty kidneys can't completely filter out of your body. Those lingering toxins damage your kidneys even more, as well as other organs. Vegetarian sources of protein are far safer for kidneys. Even becoming a part-time vegetarian naturally helps you limit your protein consumption.

Tip 6 — Sugar is Not Sweet

Added sugar in any of its numerous forms can be addictive and disease-causing, particularly when it is consumed in excess. It appears to escalate kidney damage, as well as result in obesity, diabetes, metabolic syndrome, fatty liver disease, and high blood pressure—all kidney killers. Artificial sweeteners are no better and are known nerve toxins. Satisfy your sweet tooth with fresh or frozen fruit. The fiber in fruit is a sugar controller.

Also, stop slurping soft drinks. While you're at it, eliminate all sweetened or diet beverages. They are just plain bad for you, offering no nutritional value. These disasters are consistently tied to increased risk of kidney damage, as well as risk of nearly every other known disease. Not even one a day as your "little treat" is safe. That daily soft drink is linked to a substantially greater likelihood of developing CKD and having the dreaded disease progress.

Tip 7 — Control Cholesterol

High cholesterol is linked to CKD progression and is a risk factor for cardiovascular disease. By switching what you eat from the SAD diet to a produce-centered one, you may see improvement in kidney function, lowered blood pressure, and reduced heart disease risk.

Tip 8 — Break a Sweat

Yuck, we know. But getting that blood pumping is great for the kidneys and the heart. Studies show that physically active kidney patients live longer, have fewer cardiovascular ailments, and reduce proteinuria when compared to their couch-potato counterparts.

Tip 9 — Lose Weight

Sure you're tired of that advice, but it means something when it comes to kidney health. Being overweight, particularly obese, and not eating a healthy diet are highly predictive of the development and progression of CKD. Obesity is tied to persistent protein in the urine, a sign of developing and advancing CKD. The obese progress to end stage (needing dialysis) twice as fast as normal-weight people.

Tip 10 — NO, and NO Again, to Smoking

Smoking is extremely destructive to both kidney and heart health. Smoking is significantly associated with damaged kidney function. Nicotine raises blood pressure, which also damages kidneys. Smoking increases likelihood of worsening proteinuria, and smokers progress to end stage and the need for dialysis at double the speed of non-smokers.

Part 3
Smoothie Basics

Smoothies are perfect additions to your everyday food choices, particularly as you take charge of your own health to improve kidney and heart status. Amazing is how these blended delights can be so simple and quick to make, while being so nutritious, delicious, and health-promoting. You don't need much to create perfect kidney-friendly smoothies. Just grab your blender, your favorite produce, a little liquid, and you're on your way to better health.

Chapter 6: Smoothie Tips

You'll soon become creative with your smoothie ingredients as you realize and enjoy the health benefits of these little wonders. A few points about blending and the ingredients you choose are worth considering, though, particularly if you are new at smoothie making.

Ignore "All Natural" Claims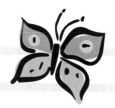

You'll reach a point where you will become creative in your smoothie ingredients, adding little extras. When selecting these extras for smoothies or for regular meals, avoid being swayed by claims of "natural" or "all natural" on food packaging. Manufacturers plaster the nearly worthless claim on both nutritious and hardly-counts-as-food items to give you the impression you're choosing an item that is as wholesome and unadulterated as if it had just been harvested.

In reality, a product labeled as natural could be healthful or a concoction from hell's kitchen. Yes, the ingredients may be "natural," but so are arsenic, hemlock, and your dog's poop. You wouldn't eat those (we hope). Carefully read the ingredients listed on the food label to know for sure whether the product is worth putting into your body.

Juicing

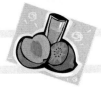

Juicing is all the rage. A growing number of juicing books pops up daily on Amazon. So, you probably wonder why this book doesn't offer juicing recipes? The answer is easy—FIBER.

Fiber is critical for control of blood sugar, lowering blood pressure, keeping your gut working properly, and lessening kidney and heart disease risks. (Revisit the earlier section on "Fiber" to refresh your memory about its health benefits).

Juicing is a process that removes fiber. Perfectly nutritious whole fruits and vegetables are placed into a juicer, which itself is expensive, and the juices of those produce items are extracted. Left behind to toss out (or to use for nutritious compost— nutrition you're no longer getting) are the fiber, protein, and numerous other antioxidants and phytochemicals accompanying the pulp.

Sure, the juice is filled with nutrients, but also with the natural sugars of the plant that are no longer tempered by the fiber. (Oh, feel the sugar rush). Eating one apple can be satisfying and is only about 60 calories. Juicing one apple gives you only 3 or 4 ounces of juice. So, you juice a couple more apples for a full serving of fiberless juice. The calories add up, the sugar rushes to your bloodstream, and you won't even feel full.

The smoothie-making process removes nothing. You get the entire edible plant item with all of its fiber, antioxidants, protein, and other nutrients. A smoothie can be quite filling and with far fewer calories than juice.

> *I juice on occasion because I enjoy the flavor of the freshly-squeezed fruit and vegetable juices. However, I use the juice as the liquid base for my fiber-filled smoothies.*

Organic vs. Conventional

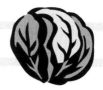

Should you buy organic fruits and vegetables for your smoothies or just use non-organic (conventional) produce? It depends.

You may recall reading about a 2012 study conducted by researchers at Stanford University.[1] They looked at 237 studies that had compared the nutritional values of organically and conventionally grown foods, and they concluded that organic foods didn't offer significant benefits over conventionally grown foods. The media jumped right on it with headlines like "Organics May Not Be Worth It."

However, the study only looked at a few vitamins and minerals and did not compare the 4,000+ antioxidants in produce or consider the effects of pesticides. Pesticides can cause cancer, nerve damage, and other health conditions. We buy organic produce specifically to avoid those toxins. The study did note that 38% of conventional produce contained detectable pesticides compared to only 7% of organics.

Obviously, organic produce is more expensive. It makes little sense to spend the extra cash on organic pineapples or bananas, as they have thick skins you probably won't eat, and such fruits aren't known to be highly contaminated.

On the other hand, strawberries and peaches consistently make the Environmental Working Group's (EWG) **Dirty Dozen** list. Check it out at ewg.org/foodnews.[2] The EWG monitors foods for pesticide exposure and reports annually the 12 most contaminated fruits and vegetables and the 15 cleanest. We use these lists for determining our organic purchases. Here are the 2014 lists:

Dirty Dozen

apples, celery, cherry tomatoes, cucumbers, grapes, hot peppers, nectarines (imported), peaches, potatoes, spinach, strawberries, sweet bell peppers, dark green lettuces (kale, collard greens), summer squash

Clean 15

asparagus, avocados, cabbage, cantaloupe, sweet corn, eggplant, grapefruit, kiwi, mangos, mushrooms, onions, papayas, pineapples, sweet peas (frozen), sweet potatoes

Caution with Dietary Supplements

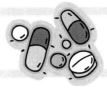

Some smoothie pros like to slip supplements into their smoothies, believing the extras will provide special boosts of energy or unique health benefits. Our smoothie recipes stay away from vitamin/mineral supplements, herbs on the National Kidney Foundation's "hit list," and protein powders for stages 1-4 of kidney disease. Here is why:

Dietary supplements, including vitamins, minerals, and certain herbs can be harmful to kidneys, especially in someone with kidney disease. More than half of U.S. adults take supplements, most taking them every day and for prolonged periods.[1]

Studies link vitamin and mineral supplements to increased risk of early death, cancer, and cardiovascular disease.[2] Most supplements don't seem to deliver their purported health benefits.

Take calcium, for example. Some 70 percent of older women and 50 percent of men take calcium pills, hoping to strengthen bones. Recent evidence suggests that getting calcium from pills may not be safe or effective. Calcium supplements may boost heart attack risk, accelerate calcification in vessels, raise likelihood of kidney stones, and increase risk of death in kidney patients.[3]

Also, multivitamins and supplements of vitamin B6, folic acid, magnesium, zinc, copper, and especially iron are all associated with greater risk of early death.[4] In view of these and similar studies, the U.S. Preventive Services Task Force now recommends against the use of supplements, including calcium.[5]

The best place to get your vitamins and minerals is straight from wholesome food, like fruits, vegetables, nuts/seeds, whole grains. As the stated in the 2010 Dietary Guidelines for Americans:

> A fundamental premise of the Dietary Guidelines is that nutrients should come primarily from food....[6]

Think about it: Isolating a single vitamin or mineral from food and taking it in pill form is absolutely nothing like eating the food itself. The whole food contains hundreds of antioxidants, phytochemicals, enzymes, and a host of other substances that work together as a team to provide health benefits. A pill of only one of those many nutrients can't realistically do the job.

Herbs

The National Kidney Foundation lists 37 herbal supplements as potentially harmful in CKD (See tables on next page).[7] One out of seven CKD patients takes at least one supplement containing an herb on the hit lists.[8]

Herbs that may be toxic to the kidneys

Artemisia absinthium (wormwood plant), Periwinkle, Autumn crocus, Sassafras, Chuifong tuokuwan (Black Pearl), Tung shueh, Horse chestnut, Vandelia cordifolia

Herbs that may be harmful in chronic kidney disease

Alfalfa,	Buckthorn	Ginger	Nettle	Vervain
Aloe	Capsicum	Ginseng	Noni juice	
Bayberry	Cascara	Horsetail	Panax	
Blue Cohosh	Coltsfoot	Licorice	Rhubarb	
Broom	Dandelion	Mate	Senna	

Herbs known to be unsafe for all people

Chapparal	Pennyroyal
Comfrey	Pokeroot
Ephedra (Ma Huang)	Sassafras
Lobelia	Senna
Mandrake	Yohimbe

People with or at risk for kidney disease are particularly vulnerable to the harmful effects of supplement use through direct toxicity to kidneys and because of decreased ability to clear the substances from their bodies, which results in excess accumulation. Some herbs increase blood pressure and worsen glycemic control, both a threat to kidneys. Some herbs trigger albuminuria and urinary tract cancer, and others interfere with medications.[9]

Major Caution

Please, never consume star fruit. The fruit is now grown in parts of the U.S., as well as in Southeast Asia. It is dangerous to already-impaired kidneys. The problem appears to be the high levels of oxalic acid in star fruit. Defective kidneys can't clear the toxic acid from the system, and within hours the excess can cause hiccups, nausea, vomiting, mental confusion, convulsions, and the need for dialysis.[10]

Protein Powders

Most kidney patients in stage 1-4 of CKD obtain too much protein from their ordinary diets, which is damaging to kidneys. So, the smoothies designed for pre-dialysis patients will not include protein powders. However, dialysis patients often suffer from undernourishment and malnutrition and require extra protein. Adding protein to their smoothies is a good way to help address the inadequacy.

The bottom line: Talk with your doctor and renal dietition about whether you need supplements (including herbs), and then only take the ones prescribed for a specific medical condition.

Blender Layering

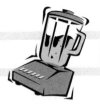

Most smoothie-makers like using a high-speed blender. It blends thoroughly and produces a thick, creamy shake.

I use an inexpensive, 2-cup blender from Target. Because it is not high-speed, my smoothies come out slightly chunky on occasion, but I like that. The little bit of chewing I must do prompts digestive juices in the mouth to begin the digestive process. I use a wide "smoothie straw."

You'll soon figure out the best way to layer your smoothie ingredients for the quickest and easiest blending. We suggest placing the liquid and juiciest fruits in the blender first. After blending those items, add the harder-to-blend ingredients (diced apple, celery, nuts), and blend again. Finally, add any leafy items (spinach, lettuce) and finish blending.

Chapter 7: Why Smoothies?

Kidney-friendly smoothies are fantastic for people trying to avoid kidney disease or who already suffer from it and hope to slow or stop its progression. Smoothies are also appropriate for individuals concerned about heart health, which should be every kidney patient. Here are a few of the many reasons to enjoy daily smoothies.

Great for Kidneys

No foods are better for kidney health than fruits and vegetables. Diets high in produce seem to decrease proteinuria, a harsh sign of progressing kidney disease, and help preserve kidney function. Fruits and vegetables help neutralize acidosis so common in kidney patients. Individuals who consume diets high in fruits and vegetables (rather than diets filled with soft drinks, red meat, fast food) are quite simply less likely to develop kidney disease and the other health conditions commonly associated with kidney disease. Your kidneys just may be what you eat.

Kidney-friendly smoothies are naturally low in harmful sodium and cholesterol and deliver no bad fats. Their ingredients are mother-nature approved, helping to lower uric acid, GFR, proteinuria, and risks for kidney stones and urinary tract infections.

Nutrient Packed

Our kidney-loving, heart-caressing smoothies are loaded with the nutritional goodness of fruits, vegetables, nuts/seeds, and whole grains. The blended result promotes kidney, heart, and overall health with impressive doses of nutrient dense goodness. Each smoothie delivers scores of disease-squashing antioxidants, enzymes, phytochemicals, fiber, vitamins, minerals—a total package of the magic available only in real food. No pill can substitute for the team of nutrients existing naturally in produce.

Our Kind of Fast Food

Do you have a couple of minutes? Few meals are more healthful or easy to prepare than a health-promoting smoothie. You certainly can't make the trip for fast food as quickly as you can whip up a smoothie wonder. Plus, smoothies provide real food rather than the disease time bomb carried into your body by fast food or processed, packaged foods. Each smoothie is great tasting, easy to digest, filling but not heavy, and the simplest way to a healthier, more energetic you. And let's not forget cleanup. Just a rinse of your blender and you're out of the kitchen.

Encourages Breakfast

A fast and fresh smoothie is the easy solution for a breakfast avoider. The nutrient-dense breakfast kick-starts the morning after the night's fast and helps you stay focused and alert throughout the day. A healthy breakfast keeps insulin levels steady all morning and prevents overeating later on. Skipping breakfast increases risk for heart disease, type 2 diabetes, and obesity.[1]

One-Mug Wonder

Smoothies become comfort food—a go-to quickie—an enjoyable and complete meal in a glass. Kidney patients often find eating burdensome and food unappetizing. A good smoothie can transform the unappetizing into a palatable delight. You will find your favorites, and return to them like old friends. While a bit of extra apple, a handful of greens, the citrus zest of a lemon may be too much to handle on a plate, the blended result often becomes an enjoyable source of energy and nutrition in an easy-to-digest shake. The well-chosen smoothie can replace a meal or provide a snack without the heavy, bloated feeling of eating too much.

Wakes Up Taste Buds

If you've consumed the typical standard American diet (SAD) for some time—sweet drinks, hamburgers, processed meats, fatty fries, and packaged, processed meals—your tongue has forgotten the joy of freshness. The pleasure and vibrance of seasonal fruits and vegetables will leave your taste buds stimulated, bringing relief from the fatty, salty coating left by SAD food.

Automatically Limits Protein

Excess protein, particularly from meat, is harsh on kidney function, and most pre-dialysis kidney patients consume way too much of the wrong kind of protein. Kidney-friendly smoothies are vegetarian based, providing the sort of protein kidneys handle better.[2] By substituting that breakfast bacon or that later-day hamburger for a smoothie, you bring yourself closer to an appropriate protein intake for kidney protection.

Treats the Whole Body

Whether you worry about kidney disease, obesity, diabetes, hypertension, heart disease, high cholesterol, cancer, or other health conditions, good nutrition is part of the answer. These one-drink wonders are an efficient way to realize health-enhancing benefits in concentrated form.

Filled with Fiber

Fiber does so many good things for our bodies, and most of us don't come near getting enough each day. The fiber in these well-balanced smoothies helps control the release of natural sugars into the blood and might help decrease the internal inflammation resulting from kidney disease.[3] Some smoothies supply nearly all of your daily fiber needs in a single glass.

Sharable

Double the recipe and share with your child, spouse, or friend. The nutritional bang of a superfood smoothie deserves to be shared. Why not take advantage of nature's sweetest nutritional bounty to show someone you're thinking of them and wishing them continued good health.

Just Plain Fun

These vibrant shakes of goodness can be enjoyed at any time by even the pickiest of eaters with special dietary needs. They can be carted anywhere, which is really great with our busy schedules. Everyone loves a good smoothie. It's even better when the smoothie is guilt free, like these.

Kid Friendly

Many kids refuse to eat vegetables on a plate, but those same veggies can be tucked into a smoothie without detection by our little, picky eaters. Several of the smoothies here are kid creations, so we know they pass the taste test for appropriate sweetness and lack of "yuck." Try several of them with your child, and feel good about providing health-promoting, concentrated nutrition rather than the sugary, salty, fatty, disease-promoting options kids tend to choose.

Gives You Bragging Rights

Yep, bragging rights. Put aside that you are doing something good for yourself by substituting super nutrition in shake form for disease-triggering meals. Put aside that you are taking real steps toward improving your overall health and helping your kidneys. Put aside that you are asserting control over your own health by choosing to put goodness into your body rather than the stuff most others consume. By enjoying your smoothies, you shift your diet toward one weighted with fruits and vegetables. That means you are on your way to becoming a vegetarian! So, brag (and we suggest you do so with self-righteousness—show some attitude).

Studies indicate that vegetarians, on average, weight less and have lower blood pressure and cholesterol than meat eaters. Vegetarians have lower risks for kidney disease, diabetes, heart disease, some cancers, and multiple other conditions. Vegetarians seem to live longer.

So, be a food snob. You are not last year's model anymore. You are becoming a new and improved you.

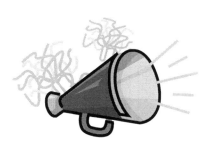

Part 4 Smoothies for Most

Part 4 includes single-serving, kidney-loving smoothies for folks who:

- ✓ *Want to avoid kidney (and heart) disease.*
- ✓ *Have kidney disease and hope to slow its progression.*
- ✓ *Want to lose weight, control diabetes, or lower blood pressure.*
- ✓ *Wish to protect a transplanted kidney.*
- ✓ *Donated a kidney or otherwise have a single kidney.*
- ✓ *Just want better health.*

Smoothies in this section are appropriate for most people (including kids) with stages 1 through 4 of chronic kidney disease. (If you were told to reduce your potassium intake, you'll want to check out smoothies in Parts 5 and 6 of this book). Phosphorus levels in Part 4 smoothies are usually modest; however, if you are unsure about a recipe, please check with your renal dietitian or go to the smoothies in Parts 5 and 6. Protein levels in Part 4 smoothies are always modest.

Cherries + Fiber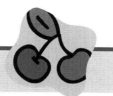

This fiber-packed beauty contains nutrients known for their ability to help regulate glucose levels, thereby offering protection from diabetes, the leading cause of kidney disease. Anthocyanins (phytonutrients) in the tasty cherries may fight destructive inflammation so common in kidney patients. Cherries also contain citrate, shown to reduce uric acid blood levels for lowered risks of gout and acidosis.

- 1 cup frozen dark cherries, unsweetened
- 1 cup banana, sliced
- 1/4 cup oat flakes (we use old-fashioned oats, right out of the container)
- 2 T. ground flax seeds
- 1 cup unsweetened, vanilla almond milk (we use Silk brand, calcium fortified)
- 1/4 tsp. cinnamon

Place all ingredients into blender and mix until smooth.

 A 2003 animal study found that substituting flaxseed meal for animal protein decreased proteinuria and renal abnormalities.[1] A 2012 study also saw improvement in kidney disease with flax use.[2]

Nutrient Values				
	Calories	414	Potassium	1102 mg
	Fat	11 g	Phosphorus	259 mg
	Fiber	14 g	Sodium	157 mg
	Protein	10 g	Calcium	526 mg

Green Tea + Peaches

After water, unsweetened green tea is the world's best drink. It's teaming with polyphenols, nutrients with multiple health benefits. Heart-healthy omega fats in walnuts help lower risk of cardiovascular disease, including hypertension. Low-fat dairy is also shown to ease blood pressure. Antioxidants in fruit can help decrease CKD-associated risks, such as inflammation and cancer.

- 1 cup freshly brewed green tea, cooled
- 1/2 single-serve container plain, nonfat Greek yogurt (3 ounces)
- 1 cup frozen peach slices, unsweetened
- 1/4 cup raw walnut halves or pieces
- 1/4 tsp. ground nutmeg

Place all ingredients into blender and mix until smooth.

A study of green tea and its effects on health showed that green tea's polyphenols could help protect kidneys from damage caused by oxidative stress.[3] Oxidative stress is involved in nearly all CKD. Talk with your doctor about drinking green tea regularly. We drink a pot (4 cups) each day.

Nutrient Values				
	Calories	305	Potassium	571 mg
	Fat	20 g	Phosphorus	248 mg
	Fiber	4 g	Sodium	35 mg
	Protein	15 g	Calcium	136 mg

Strawberry-Watermelon Mojito

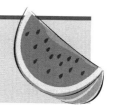

This sweet and delightful smoothie features strawberries, which are high in potassium and fiber for blood pressure control and heart health, and watermelon, which is rich in antioxidants, vitamins, and minerals and well known as kidney friendly. Basil is a powerhouse of antioxidants.

1 cup frozen strawberries, unsweetened
1 1/2 cup fresh watermelon, diced
1 T. fresh lemon juice
2 fresh basil leaves
1/4 cup water (darn, it's not rum)

Place all ingredients into your blender; mix until slushy. We enjoy this smoothie as a refreshing afternoon snack.

Heart disease, the leading cause of death in kidney patients, retreats a step with this smoothie. Researchers tracked the diets of 93,600 women and found that those who ate more than three servings of strawberries and blueberries per week were 32% less likely to have a heart attack.[4] The antioxidants and phytochemicals in the fruits seem to make blood vessels more flexible, which lowers blood pressure.

Nutrient Values	Calories	125	Potassium	504 mg
	Fat	1 g	Phosphorus	47 mg
	Fiber	5 g	Sodium	5 mg
	Protein	2 g	Calcium	43 mg

Dates to the Rescue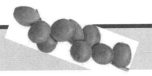

The stars of this smoothie fight disease-causing internal inflammation common in kidney patients. Those sweet dates are a good source of dietary fiber and antioxidants, as well as 15 minerals, 23 types of amino acids, and at least six vitamins. Raspberries and walnuts are fiber leaders, with free-radical-fighting antioxidants.

> 1 cup coconut milk, unsweetened (we use Blue Diamond brand)
> 2 fresh Madjool dates, chopped
> 1 cup frozen raspberries, unsweetened
> 1/4 cup raw walnut halves or pieces
> 1/4 tsp. ground cinnamon

Place the liquid and dates into a high-powered blender, mixing until smooth. Add the remaining ingredients, blending to desired consistency.

In animal studies, dates protect kidneys from toxins and inhibit cell-damaging oxidative stress that can lead to or worsen disease.[5] Eating a date is like eating candy, but without the guilt of added sugars.

Nutrient Values	Calories	435	Potassium	785 mg
	Fat	23 g	Phosphorus	182 mg
	Fiber	15 g	Sodium	127 mg
	Protein	8 g	Calcium	552 mg

Spencer's Almond-Cherry Attack

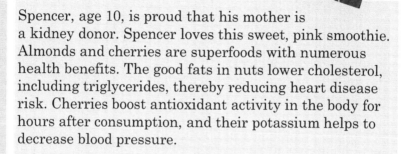

Spencer, age 10, is proud that his mother is a kidney donor. Spencer loves this sweet, pink smoothie. Almonds and cherries are superfoods with numerous health benefits. The good fats in nuts lower cholesterol, including triglycerides, thereby reducing heart disease risk. Cherries boost antioxidant activity in the body for hours after consumption, and their potassium helps to decrease blood pressure.

1 cup unsweetened almond milk
1 cup frozen, dark red cherries, unsweetened
1/4 cup raw almond slivers
1/4 tsp. almond extract
1/2 tsp. vanilla extract

Place all ingredients into blender and mix until smooth.

A late 2012 study found that consuming cherries within the previous two days lowered risk of a gout attack by 35% compared to not eating cherries.[6] The antioxidants in cherries reduce serum uric acid levels to decrease inflammation and provide kidney protection.

Nutrient Values	Calories	289	Potassium	578 mg
	Fat	16 g	Phosphorus	182 mg
	Fiber	7 g	Sodium	150 mg
	Protein	8 g	Calcium	543 mg

Pear + Pineapple

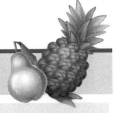

This pale green potion contains an impressive amount of fiber for weight control and better health. Pineapple is shown to speed healing, and the heart-healthy fats in avocado may help lower the all-too-common heart disease risk in kidney disease.

1/2 cup 100% orange juice, calcium fortified.
1 cup frozen pineapple chunks, unsweetened
1/2 medium fresh pear with peel, seeded and diced
1/4 fresh avocado, peeled
1/4 cup oat flakes (we use old fashioned oats)
1/2 tsp. ground cinnamon

Place all ingredients into your blender, and mix until smooth. Add a little water for a thinner consistency.

Metabolic syndrome (MS) refers to the presence of several cardiovascular risk factors in the same person (see P. 16) MS raises risk of CKD by nearly three times. In a study involving 26,000 patients with stage 3 or 4 CKD, 60% had MS. During the 3 year study, 48% of MS patients reached end stage, needing dialysis. Those with MS were 30% more likely to die during the study than kidney patients without MS.[7] Changing your diet can lower risk of MS.

Nutrient Values				
	Calories	360	Potassium	871 mg
	Fat	10 g	Phosphorus	159 mg
	Fiber	12 g	Sodium	7 mg
	Protein	7 g	Calcium	298 mg

Sully's Virgin Pina Colada

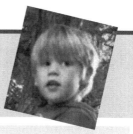

An inherited form of kidney disease runs in Sullivan's family, and so far this 4-year-old is CKD free. Sully loves fruit smoothies, and this trilogy of health-promoting pineapple, strawberries, and bananas is his favorite. Coconut milk adds an unbeatable richness and flavor.

- 1 cup coconut milk, unsweetened (we use Blue Diamond brand)
- 1/4 cup frozen pineapple chunks, unsweetened
- 1/2 cup banana slices
- 1/2 cup frozen strawberries, unsweetened

Place all ingredients into blender and mix until smooth.

Unexpected events can cause kidney function measures to fluctuate. Researchers compared 64 diabetic kidney patients with healthy adults. Subjects ate 44 g. protein in the form of either 2 quarter-pounders or 2 veggie burgers. Stage 3 kidney patients had a significant drop in kidney function measures just hours after eating the meat, compared to the veggie burger eaters who saw no decline.[8]

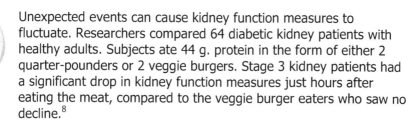

Nutrient Values	Calories	159	Potassium	873 mg
	Fat	4 g	Phosphorus	44 mg
	Fiber	5 g	Sodium	128 mg
	Protein	2 g	Calcium	472 mg

Experimenting with Kale

This ultra-healthy smoothie is antioxidant-rich. Kale is high in calcium and fiber and has 45 different flavonoids and dozens of phytonutrients to fight nasty free radicals roaming in a kidney patient's body. Kale is also loaded with vitamin K, and a serving contains over 5 times the recommended daily allowance.

1 cup water or freshly brewed green tea, cooled
1/2 cup fresh or frozen pineapple chunks, unsweetened
1 cup frozen blackberries, unsweetened
1/4 avocado, peeled
1/2 tsp. fresh ginger root, chopped
1/2 cup firmly packed raw kale, chopped and center stem removed

Place all ingredients except the kale into blender and mix until smooth. Add the kale, blending to desired consistency.

Emerging research indicates that vitamin K (in leafy greens) may help prevent and treat vascular calcification (calcium build-up in vessels) in kidney patients.[9] Vascular calcification hardens arteries, causing heart attacks, strokes, and early death. In kidney disease, calcium is often leached from bones and deposited in vessels as kidney function deteriorates.

Nutrient Values	Calories	247	Potassium	763 mg
	Fat	9 g	Phosphorus	114 mg
	Fiber	14 g	Sodium	21 mg
	Protein	6 g	Calcium	116 mg

Kit's Indian/Thai Inspiration

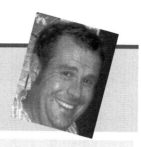

Kit is administrator of our www.kidneysteps.com website and loves creating exotic smoothies. This unusual treat stresses healthful turmeric; antioxidant-rich mangos to reduce inflammation in kidney disease; and cardamom, often used to treat mild stomach and intestinal distress. Nuts provide heart-healthy fats to lower cardiovascular risk. Who could resist this breakfast feast?

- 1 cup coconut milk, unsweetened (we use Blue Diamond brand)
- 1 cup frozen mango cubes, unsweetened
- 2 T. 100% cashew butter, unsweetened and unsalted
- 1 tsp. ground turmeric
- 2 green cardamom pods

Place all ingredients into blender and mix until smooth. If this smoothie is too tart for you, Kit suggests adding 5 drops liquid stevia or 1/2 teaspoon agave.

Adults who eat nuts and nut butters are less likely to have hypertension and LDL (bad) cholesterol, according to a well-publicized study. Individuals (2,450 of them) followed a low-fat diet, and 4,997 followed a Mediterranean diet (similar to DASH), having either olive oil or nuts each day. At follow-up, the olive oil/nut eaters were 40% less likely to suffer a stroke than the low-fat dieters and 30% less likely to have a heart attack or die of heart disease during the study.[10]

Nutrient Values	Calories	353	Potassium	716 mg
	Fat	20 g	Phosphorus	192 mg
	Fiber	7 g	Sodium	133 mg
	Protein	8 g	Calcium	487 mg

Touch of Thyme

In studies, blueberries are shown to help prevent urinary tract infections, reduce blood pressure, improve memory and mood, and promote healthy aging. Thyme helps neutralize bugs, including strains of *E. coli* and staph that cause serious illness. Low-fat dairy also helps reduce blood pressure. This smoothie provides it all.

1/2 cup nonfat milk
1/2 single serving container nonfat, plain Greek yogurt (3 ounces)
1/2 cup banana slices
1 cup frozen blueberries, unsweetened (we like organic wild blueberries)
1/2 tsp. fresh thyme leaves (removed from stem)
2 T. raw sunflower seeds

Place all ingredients into blender and mix until smooth. Add additional liquid as needed to blend to desired consistency.

One of five kidney patients suffers from depression, even in early CKD. In an analysis of 25 studies that included 2,000 men followed for about 13 years, adherence to a healthy diet, as opposed to a Western or Japanese diet, was associated with a lower prevalence of depressive symptoms and decreased risk of depression. A healthy diet was characterized by berries and other fruits, vegetables, whole grains, low-fat dairy, and fish.[11]

Nutrient Values				
	Calories	341	Potassium	789 mg
	Fat	10 g	Phosphorus	389 mg
	Fiber	10 g	Sodium	89 mg
	Protein	18 g	Calcium	287 mg

Clara's Fruit 'n' Veggies

Clara's mother, grandmother, and two aunts have kidney disease. So far, young Clara is fine. Clara regularly drinks smoothies containing nutrient-dense vegetables, along with fruit and protein. The variety of antioxidants and phytochemicals boosts good health.

1/2 cup soy milk, unsweetened
1/2 cup banana, sliced
1/2 single-serving container nonfat, plain Greek yogurt (3 ounces)
1/4 cup carrots, sliced
1/4 cup frozen green peas
1/2 cup frozen strawberries, unsweetened

Place all ingredients into blender and mix until smooth.

Unfolding research suggests that vitamin D, a hormone, may work miracles. Vitamin D deficiency is linked to increased risks for cancer, depression, dementia, gum disease, hypertension, faster progression of CKD, and early failure of a transplanted kidney. Researchers recently studied 101 CKD patients not on dialysis and with albuminuria. Half the patients received a vitamin D analogue daily. After six months, albuminuria in these patients dropped nearly in half and their parathyroid hormone fell by 14%, compared to patients not taking vitamin D. Researchers concluded that the vitamin D analogue can slow progression of kidney disease and relieve hyperparathyroidism common in CKD.[12]

Nutrient Values				
	Calories	233	Potassium	742 mg
	Fat	3 g	Phosphorus	232 mg
	Fiber	6 g	Sodium	148 mg
	Protein	15 g	Calcium	278 mg

Peach Milkshake for "D"

Yes, this peach milkshake smoothie may improve heart health and cholesterol with the good fats in walnuts, the fiber of oatmeal, and the cholesterol-busting cinnamon. But, let's focus on the vitamin D supplied by dairy because an association exists between vitamin D, kidney disease, and albuminuria (see below).

1 cup skim milk (fortified with vitamin D)
1 cup frozen peach slices, unsweetened
1/4 cup oat flakes (we use old fashioned oats)
2 T. raw walnut pieces
1/2 teas. ground cinnamon
1/2 teas. pure vanilla extract
pinch of ground nutmeg

Place all ingredients into blender and mix until smooth.

Vitamin D deficiency is prominent in kidney patients and is clearly associated with kidney disease. Researchers found that people deficient in vitamin D were 70% more likely to have albuminuria (protein in urine), a prime indicator of kidney disease.[13] Sunlight and dairy are primary vitamin D sources.

Nutrient Values				
Calories	325	Potassium	821 mg
Fat	12 g	Phosphorus	413 mg
Fiber	6 g	Sodium	104 mg
Protein	15 g	Calcium	347 mg

UTI and Stone Aid

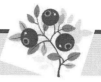

Urinary tract infections and kidney stones are not only painful but can also result in kidney disease. Cranberries are traditionally used to fight off both. This pink beauty is also high in antioxidants to reduce cardiovascular risks, internal inflammation, and acidosis.

1/2 cup 100% cranberry juice, unsweetened
1/2 cup navel orange segments
1 cup frozen banana slices (freeze in advance)
1 tsp. orange zest (zest orange before peeling)
1/4 cup raw walnuts, halves or pieces
1/2 tsp. ground cinnamon

Place all ingredients into blender and mix until smooth. Add a little water for a thinner consistency.

Despite some debate, recent research supports that cranberries may be effective in preventing UTIs by stopping *E. coli* from sticking to other bacteria in the bladder, thus making it easier to flush them from the urinary tract.[14] Also, cranberry juice lowers the pH of urine, making acidic urine alkaline, which helps prevent formation of kidney stones.[15]

Nutrient Values				
	Calories	428	Potassium	910 mg
	Fat	20 g	Phosphorus	170 mg
	Fiber	10 g	Sodium	7 mg
	Protein	8 g	Calcium	98 mg

Pumpkin + Banana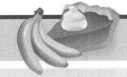

Besides its deep orange loveliness, pumpkin contains kidney-friendly beta-carotene shown to help promote healthy skin and may even prevent premature wrinkling. Banana and nuts offer loads of potassium to help lower blood pressure. Oats, of course, are heart healthy, which also means kidney healthy.

1/2 cup soy milk, unsweetened
1/4 cup 100% pumpkin puree (not pumpkin pie filling)
1/2 cup banana slices, frozen in advance
1 T. 100% peanut butter, unsalted
1/4 cup oat flakes (straight from a box of old-fashioned oats)
1/2 tsp. cinnamon

Place all ingredients into blender and mix until smooth. Add more soy milk if you prefer a thinner consistency.

Added sugars--real or artificial--may just cause many kidney disease cases. Researchers reviewed studies about the issue and found significant associations between added sugar and increased uric acid levels, diabetes, obesity, proteinuria, and increased risk of kidney damage and disease.[16] Kidney-friendly smoothies offer a naturally sweet option to added sugars.

Nutrient Values	Calories	314	Potassium	725 mg
	Fat	12 g	Phosphorus	231 mg
	Fiber	8 g	Sodium	65 mg
	Protein	12 g	Calcium	200 mg

Valentine Smoothie

This smoothie is kidney love in a glass and deserves attention on "heart" day. The rich flavonoids of dark chocolate may aid in decreasing blood pressure and cholesterol levels. While research is ongoing, coffee's antioxidants just might lower risks for hypertension, heart disease, and diabetes.

1/2 cup brewed coffee, cooled
1/2 cup vanilla almond milk, unsweetened
1 cup frozen dark cherries, unsweetened
1 tsp. dark cocoa powder, unsweetened
    (at least 60% cacao)
2 T. raw almond slivers
1/4 tsp. ground cinnamon
1 tsp. honey

Place all ingredients into blender and mix until smooth. Reduce the almond milk if you want a thicker treat.

Hypertension causes kidney disease, and kidney disease causes hypertension—a vicious cycle. The ingredients in this smoothie may aid in controlling blood pressure. In an analysis of 20 studies, flavanol-rich chocolate and cocoa showed a significant blood-pressure lowering effect.[17] Likewise, a large French retrospective analysis of 176,437 people tied coffee and tea consumption to lowered blood pressure.[18]

Nutrient Values				
	Calories	241	Potassium	557 mg
	Fat	9 g	Phosphorus	126 mg
	Fiber	6 g	Sodium	78 mg
	Protein	6 g	Calcium	287 mg

Salad in a Glass

This is our version of V-8 for kidneys and delivers nearly 4 servings of vegetables. Research shows that consuming vegetables just might be one of the best things you can do for better health. Think of the antioxidants, vitamins, minerals, and enzymes in this low-calorie delight. Olive oil is great for the heart, blood pressure, and cholesterol; and garlic fights infections.

1/2 cup water or crushed ice
1/2 cup fresh tomato, diced
1/4 cup cucumber, diced
1/4 cup red pepper, chopped
1/4 cup celery, chopped
1 cup red leaf lettuce, chopped
2 tsp. fresh chives, chopped
1/2 clove fresh garlic, minced
1 tsp. extra virgin olive oil
1 tsp. fresh lemon juice

Place all ingredients into blender and mix until smooth. Sprinkle in some black pepper and a pinch of red pepper flakes, if you enjoy spicy like we do.

A diet high in the foods stressed in this book is tied to avoidance of CKD or slowing its progression. In a study of 2,300 people, those consuming a diet that included fruits, vegetable, nuts, low-fat dairy did not develop albuminuria at the same rate as those consuming fast food, processed meats, soft drinks. Obesity and smoking also increased CKD risk.[19]

Nutrient Values				
	Calories	84	Potassium	466 mg
	Fat	5 g	Phosphorus	57 mg
	Fiber	3 g	Sodium	33 mg
	Protein	2 g	Calcium	40 mg

Jack's Orange Dreamsicle

Jack, age 9, knows what he likes, and he likes oranges. Oranges contain a pharmacy's worth of salves for the heart. Pectin, a soluble fiber in oranges, acts like a giant sponge, sopping up cholesterol in food and blocking its absorption. Potassium in oranges and yogurt counterbalance salt, helping to keep blood pressure under control.

- 1 tsp. orange zest
- 1 medium seedless orange, peeled and sectioned
- 1/2 single serving container nonfat, plain Greek yogurt (3 ounces)
- 1/2 tsp. vanilla extract
- 1/2 tsp. cinnamon
- 1/2 cup frozen pineapple chunks, unsweetened

Place all ingredients except the pineapple into your blender, and mix until smooth. Add the pineapple, blending to make a delicious smoothie. You may need to add 1/4 cup additional liquid to blend the pineapple.

Trillions of microbes reside in our intestines, helping to digest our food and convert it to energy and fat. Developing research suggests that a healthy diet (one that includes the foods in our smoothies) may help lower obesity by encouraging leanness-related microbes to populate the gut, leading to better weight control. In contrast, the standard American diet causes obesity-related microbes to flourish.[20]

Nutrient Values				
	Calories	171	Potassium	455 mg
	Fat	1 g	Phosphorus	156 mg
	Fiber	5 g	Sodium	33 mg
	Protein	10 g	Calcium	181 mg

Ben's Fruit Creation

Ben is familiar with kidney disease because his mother is a kidney donor. At 13, Ben has mastered smoothies, and this is a go-to as he's rushing off to school. Protein in the dairy keeps him alert, and the fruit is just tasty. Ben may not realize his creation helps him stay healthy with its superfruit antioxidants and high potassium content to help counter salty food he might sneak in during the day.

1/2 cup 100% orange juice, calcium fortified
1/2 cup skim milk
1 medium banana, sliced
1 cup frozen strawberries, unsweetened
1 frozen organic, nonfat plain yogurt stick (2 ounces)

Ben places all ingredients into his personal single-serve blender, and mixes until smooth.

Tobacco use harms kidneys and raises risk of kidney disease. CKD in smokers also progresses more quickly, and smokers do worse on dialysis and after kidney transplantation. Smoking even deteriorates the quality of a donated kidney. In a review of 635 living kidney donations between 2000 and 2008, recipients receiving kidneys from smokers had a 31% greater risk of early loss of that kidney than did recipients of kidneys from non-smokers.[21]

Nutrient Values				
	Calories	317	Potassium	1,275 mg
	Fat	1 g	Phosphorus	274 mg
	Fiber	7 g	Sodium	67 mg
	Protein	13 g	Calcium	494 mg

Fun with Watermelon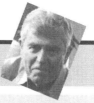

Bob (husband of co-author Vicki) isn't fond of zucchini and had never tasted chia seeds until he tried this smoothie and loved it. Watermelon is a heavyweight in the nutrient department, with a nice dose of vitamins A and C and a healthy shot of potassium and lycopene. Chia seeds are loaded with fiber, and zucchini contains vitamin C and other important antioxidants.

1 cup watermelon, cubed
1/2 cup frozen strawberries, unsweetened
1/4 cup coconut water
1/2 cup zucchini, diced
1 T. chia seeds

Place all ingredients into blender and mix until smooth.

Oral disease is common in people with CKD and stems largely from internal inflammation, poor nutrition, and lack of dental care. In a review of 88 studies, researches found that gum disease was more common as CKD progressed. One-quarter of stage 5 patients never brushed their teeth, and only 11% flossed. The state of the gums might reflect cardiovascular disease prognosis, the researchers suggested.[22]

Nutrient Values	Calories	163	Potassium	614 mg
	Fat	5 g	Phosphorus	196 mg
	Fiber	9 g	Sodium	26 mg
	Protein	5 g	Calcium	136 mg

Simply Blueberries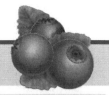

This smoothie contains kidney-friendly ingredients that may lower blood pressure and aid heart health. Blueberries and orange juice were found to help lower destructive internal inflammation, among other good attributes. Yogurt and nuts are heart-healthy and supply important protein.

1/2 cup 100% pure orange juice, calcium-fortified
1/4 cup water
1/2 single-serve container nonfat, plain Greek yogurt
   (3 ounces)
1 cup frozen blueberries, unsweetened
1/4 cup raw cashews

Place all ingredients into your blender, mixing until smooth. Add a little more water if you prefer a thinner consistency.

 Restricting protein consumption slows kidney disease progression, say researchers in a recent review of literature. They concluded that a Western diet high in animal protein (meat, cheese, fish) is acid-inducing and speeds CKD progression (lowers GFR). A plant-based diet high in fruits and vegetables is alkaline-inducing and can slow CKD progression. The researchers recommended the DASH diet to preserve kidney function, with modification as needed to reduce potassium in late-stage CKD.[23]

Nutrient Values				
	Calories	343	Potassium	649 mg
	Fat	13 g	Phosphorus	322 mg
	Fiber	7 g	Sodium	39 mg
	Protein	15 g	Calcium	378 mg

Blood Pressure Magic

Check your blood pressure before enjoying this effective smoothie and then about 6 hours later. You just might notice a drop thanks to the combination of beets and Grana Padano cheese, a parmesan cheese.

- 1/2 cup water
- 1/2 cup 100% unsweetened orange juice, fortified with calcium
- 1/4 cup raw beets, peeled and diced
- 1 cup frozen, dark cherries, unsweetened
- 2 T. Grana Padano cheese
- 1 T. ground flax seeds

Place all ingredients into blender and mix until smooth.

Research shows that integrating Grana Padano cheese into the diet of mildly hypertensive individuals not taking anti-hypertensive drugs resulted in a significant drop in mean blood pressure of 7 to 8 mmHg compared to the blood pressure of people not eating the cheese.[24] So, why not regularly substitute Grana Padano for other cheeses?

Nutrient Values				
	Calories	255	Potassium	579 mg
	Fat	10 g	Phosphorus	279 mg
	Fiber	9 g	Sodium	199 mg
	Protein	13 g	Calcium	686 mg

Bloody Mary for Health

Darn, no booze. But, this low-cal mix of over 4 vegetable servings is worth making. Parsley, basil and oregano offer a host of health benefits with their antioxidants and vitamins. Garlic can help regulate blood pressure and cholesterol and is a powerful natural antibiotic. Tomato contains lycopene, a cancer-fighting phytochemical. The heart-healthy olive oil is there to help you absorb certain nutrients in the smoothie.

1/2 cup sodium free tomato juice
1/4 cup fresh celery, diced
1/4 cup cucumber with peel, diced
1 cup fresh tomato, chopped
1/2 clove fresh garlic, chopped
1 T. fresh flat-leaf parsley, chopped
2 fresh basil leaves
4 fresh oregano leaves
1 tsp. extra virgin olive oil
1 tsp. fresh lime juice

Place all ingredients into blender and mix until smooth. We add red pepper flakes and fresh black pepper for the heat.

CKD patients often develop abnormal left heart ventricles and heart disease. Scientists had 36 CKD patients exercise 150 minutes a week (20-30 min/day) on a treadmill, stationary bike, or rowing machine and use weights twice/week. Another 36 CKD patients received their normal care. After 12 months, the exercise group improved cardiac function by 20% and the non-exercise group lost function by an additional 6%. Exercise can help you reduce risk of cardiovascular death in CKD.[25]

Nutrient Values				
	Calories	107	Potassium	856 mg
	Fat	5 g	Phosphorus	84 mg
	Fiber	4 g	Sodium	45 mg
	Protein	3 g	Calcium	68 mg

Anti-Inflammatory Snack

This pale orange smoothie is anti-inflammatory. Turmeric (curcumin) is actively studied for its kidney and other health benefits. The carotenoids of papaya are also shown to aid kidney health. Green tea, the least processed of traditional teas, provides high levels of antioxidants, polyphenols, and epigallocatechin-3-gallate (EGCG), found to be kidney- and heart-protective.

1/2 cup fresh green tea, cooled
1 cup frozen pineapple chunks
1 cup fresh papaya chunks
1/4 tsp. turmeric
1 T. ground flax seeds
1/2 tsp. fresh ginger root, grated

Place all ingredients into blender and mix until smooth. This smoothie is a pleasant afternoon snack.

CKD is characterized by a continuous reduction in kidney function and increased inflammation. This internal inflammation further accelerates kidney decline. Researchers found that turmeric (curcumin) helped reduce destructive inflammation.[26]

Nutrient Values				
	Calories	185	Potassium	535 mg
	Fat	4 g	Phosphorus	75 mg
	Fiber	7 g	Sodium	17 mg
	Protein	3 g	Calcium	71 mg

Green De-Stresser

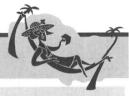

Had a difficult day? De-stress with a nutrient-rich smoothie. The folic acid helps create dopamine, a neurotransmitter associated with pleasure. Vitamin C, important to kidney patients, aids in returning blood pressure and cortical levels to normal. Veggies neutralize acidosis, and their antioxidants fight free radicals. You'll want to sit quietly as you sip this delight.

1 tsp. orange zest
1 medium naval orange, peeled and sectioned
1/2 cup 100% orange juice, calcium-fortified
1 cup baby romaine lettuce leaves, shredded
1/2 cup frozen sweet peas

Place the first three ingredients into blender and mix until smooth. Add the lettuce and frozen peas, blending well.

Within 6 months following kidney transplantation, 21% of recipients develop "new onset diabetes after transplant" (NODAT). NODAT is associated with worse outcomes and higher rates of cardiovascular disease, graft failure, and death. Lifestyle factors, particularly healthy eating, can prevent NODAT.[27] This smoothie provides 2 servings each of fruit and vegetables for NODAT prevention.

Nutrient Values	Calories	187	Potassium	702 mg
	Fat	1 g	Phosphorus	122 mg
	Fiber	8 g	Sodium	78 mg
	Protein	6 g	Calcium	344 mg

Fiber Power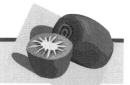

Ounce for ounce, kiwi has more vitamin C than an orange and more potassium than a banana. Kiwi also is associated with improved blood pressure. Chia seeds deliver a big dose of omega-3 fat and a host of other nutrients. Research indicates chia seeds may help to stabilize blood sugar and lower risk of cardiovascular disease. This delicious smoothie delivers at least half your fiber needs for the day, important since fiber might lower creatinine levels and improve kidney function.

1/2 cup skim milk
1 medium kiwi fruit, peeled and diced
1 cup banana slices, frozen in advance
2 T. chia seeds

Place all ingredients into blender and mix until smooth.

Dietary fiber may lower risk of early death in kidney patients, and fiber has anti-inflammatory properties. An analysis of 14,533 people showed that each 10 g/day increment in total fiber intake was associated with a 38% decreased likelihood of developing damaging inflammation markers and a 19% lowered risk of early death in people with kidney disease.[28] A recent study also showed that dietary fiber can lower creatinine levels and improve eGFR.[29]

Nutrient Values	Calories	369	Potassium	987 mg
	Fat	10 g	Phosphorus	444 mg
	Fiber	17 g	Sodium	60 mg
	Protein	11 g	Calcium	357 mg

Acai-Berry Smoothie

While acai berries top the charts in antioxidants and phytochemicals, strawberries and raspberries aren't far behind. Together, these berries are leaders at keeping your brain going and reducing risks for heart disease, diabetes, and cancer. Refreshing coconut water is high in blood pressure-lowering potassium and contains no cholesterol.

- 1 cup 100% coconut water, unsweetened (we use Naked brand)
- 1/2 cup acai berries, unsweetened
- 1/2 cup frozen strawberries, unsweetened
- 1/2 cup frozen raspberries, unsweetened
- 1/2 single-serving container plain, nonfat Greek yogurt (3 ounces)

Place all ingredients into blender and mix until smooth.

A nutritious diet might assist kidney patients with sleeping difficulties. A recent study of 44 patients in early, mid, or late stage kidney disease revealed that 53% had significant insomnia, 33% suffered from sleep apnea, and 24% showed both insomnia and apnea.[30]

Nutrient Values	Calories	226	Potassium	923 mg
	Fat	6 g	Phosphorus	191 mg
	Fiber	10 g	Sodium	295 mg
	Protein	12 g	Calcium	199 mg

Memory Smoothie

Kidney patients may notice a reduction in cognitive skills (yikes!) associated with persistent proteinuria. A combined deficiency of iron and omega-3 fatty acids might hinder long-term memory, says research. This heart-kidney-brain-healthy smoothie can help combat those nutrient deficiencies with high-fiber, iron-rich beans, flax with omega-3 fats, and loads of antioxidants. By the way, you won't even notice the beans.

1 cup water
1/3 cup black beans, cooked and unsalted
1 cup frozen dark cherries, unsweetened
1/2 cup fresh or frozen strawberries, sliced and unsweetened
2 T. ground flax seeds

Place all ingredients into blender and mix until smooth.

Can't reason as well as you once did? Kidney disease has emerged as a possible risk factor for cognitive impairment and dementia. Persistent albuminuria (protein in urine) is associated with increased risk of cognitive decline even at a relatively young age and even in earlier CKD stages.[31] Stay sharp with good nutrition.

Nutrient Values				
	Calories	277	Potassium	833 mg
	Fat	7 g	Phosphorus	226 mg
	Fiber	14 g	Sodium	7 mg
	Protein	10 g	Calcium	102 mg

Kidney Aid 101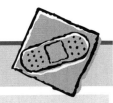

Almonds contain good fats and yogurt has live cultures, both of which may improve heart health. Blueberries, kale, and bananas are great sources of potassium, fiber, antioxidants, and multiple vitamins, important in kidney disease. Water preserves kidney function (see below).

1 cup water
1 cup frozen blueberries, unsweetened
1/2 cup banana, sliced
1 T. pure almond butter (almonds are sole ingredient on jar)
1/2 container single-serving fat-free, plain Greek yogurt (3 ounces)
1/2 cup firmly-packed kale, chopped (we often substitute arugula)

Place all ingredients except the kale into blender and mix until smooth. Add the kale, blending to desired consistency. This is a big smoothie but low-cal.

 Plain water is the best drink for kidney patients. Studies suggest a strong, direct association between preservation of kidney function and fluid intake. Benefits come from drinking 3 to 4 liters (quarts) of water per day. Increased water slows cyst growth in PKD, too.[32] Check with your nephrologist before increasing your water intake.

Nutrient Values				
	Calories	311	Potassium	767 mg
	Fat	10 g	Phosphorus	261 mg
	Fiber	11 g	Sodium	50 mg
	Protein	15 g	Calcium	228 mg

Pear-Peach-Mango Tango

Don't be fooled by the paleness of this smoothie. It sneaks in loads of antioxidants to fight cancer risk and protect cells from DNA damage. White fruits like pear and apple help reduce cholesterol and stroke risk, say studies. Chia seeds provide important fiber and protein.

1 cup almond milk, unsweetened (we use Silk brand)
1/2 fresh pear with peel, diced
1/2 cup frozen peach slices, unsweetened
1/2 cup frozen mango chunks, unsweetened
1 T. chia seeds

Place all ingredients into blender and mix until smooth.

Low-cal, nutrient dense smoothies help promote weight loss. Obesity (hello, 36% of us) is a risk factor for kidney disease, progression of CKD, and proteinuria. The obese propel to end stage and the need for dialysis twice as fast as normal weight kidney patients. Losing even a few pounds by improving diet is shown to reduce proteinuria, slow kidney disease progression, and improve heart health.[33]

Nutrient Values				
	Calories	230	Potassium	446 mg
	Fat	8 g	Phosphorus	191 mg
	Fiber	12 g	Sodium	155 mg
	Protein	5 g	Calcium	560 mg

Nausea Easer

Want to soothe a stomach? This powerful package contains ingredients found helpful in calming upset tummies. If nausea lasts more than a short time, your doctor should determine its cause.

1/2 cup water or freshly brewed green tea, cooled
1/2 cup frozen green grapes (freeze in advance)
1 cup banana slices
1 T. fresh ginger root, chopped
2 fresh peppermint leaves

Place all ingredients into blender and mix until smooth.

The National Kidney Foundation promotes ginger as kidney-friendly and helpful for nausea.[34] According to the National Library of Medicine, ginger is used worldwide for treatment of appetite loss, nausea and vomiting, stomach upset, flatulence, motion sickness, and colon inflammation.[35] Studies are mixed but confirm that ginger helps relieve mild nausea.[36]

Nutrient Values				
	Calories	191	Potassium	707 mg
	Fat	1 g	Phosphorus	50 mg
	Fiber	5 g	Sodium	5 mg
	Protein	3 g	Calcium	17 mg

Vicki's Berry Blast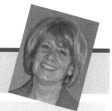

Numerous studies stress the potential health benefits of berries, thanks to their vast array of antioxidants. Anthocyanins in berries may lower blood pressure, cut heart disease risk, and are anti-inflammatory, all important in kidney disease. Walnuts and oats are shown to lower cholesterol and heart disease risk. Enjoy three daily servings of fruit, as well as the fiber and good fats in one yummy smoothie.

1/2 cup fresh (or frozen) strawberries, unsweetened
1/2 cup fresh or frozen blackberries, unsweetened
1/2 cup frozen dark cherries, unsweetened
1 tsp. lemon or orange zest
1/4 cup oat flakes (we use old-fashioned oats)
2 T. raw walnut halves or pieces
1/2 cup water

Place all ingredients into blender and mix until smooth. If using all frozen fruit, add additional water for a thinner consistency.

In a 2013 study of 66,105 women, high consumption of fruits (not juices) was associated with lowered risk of type 2 diabetes (the leading cause of kidney disease).[37] Is any fruit better than naturally sweet berries?

Nutrient Values				
	Calories	311	Potassium	462 mg
	Fat	11 g	Phosphorus	182 mg
	Fiber	12 g	Sodium	4 mg
	Protein	7 g	Calcium	69 mg

Soy-Apricot-Date Delight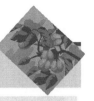

Recent studies suggest a positive link between soy and kidney protection. Apricots provide kidney-friendly beta-carotene, and berries turn on detoxifying enzymes. This smoothie combination makes a health-promoting meal.

1 cup soymilk, fortified and unsweetened
2 fresh apricots, diced and pit removed
1/2 cup frozen raspberries, unsweetened
1 Medjool date, diced and pit removed
1/4 cup frozen edamame (soy beans)

Place all ingredients into high-speed blender and mix until smooth. If using all frozen fruit, add additional water for a thinner consistency.

Researchers looked at 481 overweight/obese individuals. After six months, they saw a 25% reduction in urine protein in subjects losing just 4.2 centimeters of belly fat, and an 11% reduction in those cutting 314 mg. of phosphates from processed foods. Researchers noted that the body handles phosphates from produce better than from processed foods. To cut kidney damage, trim body fat and steer clear of processed foods.[38]

Nutrient Values				
	Calories	244	Potassium	875 mg
	Fat	6 g	Phosphorus	174 mg
	Fiber	10 g	Sodium	94 mg
	Protein	12 g	Calcium	359 mg

Green Super Shake

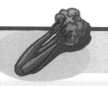

Celery and honeydew in this cool green drink act as diuretics to help rinse toxins from your system. Greens are superfoods bursting with antioxidants, vitamins, and minerals to support better kidney and overall health.

1/4 cup 100% orange juice (calcium fortified)
1 cup honeydew melon, cubed
1/2 cup frozen pineapple chunks, unsweetened
1 medium stalk of celery, diced
1/4 cup oat flakes (we use old fashioned oats)
2 fresh mint leaves, torn
1/2 cup fresh bibb lettuce, chopped (also called Boston, butterhead)

Place all ingredients into blender and mix until smooth. Add more liquid if you like a thinner consistency.

Have a pet? The AHA released its Scientific Statement in June 2013, reporting on research that found associations between pet ownership and lower blood pressure, heart rate, and cholesterol. Dog owners get more physical activity and are less likely to be overweight or to smoke, leading to better cardiovascular health. They also live longer on average than non-dog owners.[39]

Nutrient Values				
	Calories	215	Potassium	806 mg
	Fat	2 g	Phosphorus	133 mg
	Fiber	6 g	Sodium	55 mg
	Protein	5 g	Calcium	177 mg

Jennifer's Kidney Balm

Having donated one of my kidneys, I guard my remaining one by carefully watching what I eat and engaging in regular exercise. I enjoy this pale smoothie with its kidney-protective beta-carotene from the pumpkin, carrots, and pumpkin seeds. The antioxidants from the spinach are a nutritious bonus. Oxalate kidney-stone formers will want to substitute lettuce for the spinach.

- 3/4 cup unsweetened almond milk
- 1/3 cup 100% pumpkin (if using canned, buy no-salt pumpkin)
- 1/2 cup frozen carrot slices
- 2 T. unsalted pumpkin seeds
- 1 cup fresh spinach leaves

Place all ingredients into blender and mix until smooth. Add more liquid if you like a thinner consistency.

Kidneys help excrete many drugs we take, and some of those drugs can harm kidneys. A significant cause of kidney damage is long-term use of non-steroidal anti-inflammatory drugs (NSAIDs). NSAIDs include aspirin (in Bayer and Ecotrin, for example), ibuprofen (in Advil and Motrin, for example), and naproxen (in Aleve, for example). NSAIDs are also in many other prescription and non-prescription products. Children are particularly vulnerable to the toxic effects of NSAIDs. In a study of kids suffering acute kidney injury caused by NSAIDs, 75% had taken the correct dosage.[40]

Nutrient Values				
	Calories	207	Potassium	769 mg
	Fat	8 g	Phosphorus	107 mg
	Fiber	8 g	Sodium	190 mg
	Protein	8 g	Calcium	428 mg

Drinkable Sunscreen

The ingredients of this smoothie are packed with powerful phytochemicals that may help protect kidney patients from developing companion diseases such as cancer. Green tea is abundant in catechins, an antioxidant known to protect cells from cancer. Broccoli is also a known cancer-fighter.

1 cup frozen pineapple chunks, unsweetened
1/2 cup water or freshly brewed green tea, cooled
1/4 ripe avocado, peeled and diced
1/4 cup fresh or frozen broccoli
1 tsp. fresh lemon juice
1/2 cup fresh romaine leaves, chopped and firmly packed

Place all ingredients except lettuce into blender, and mix until smooth. Add the lettuce, continuing to blend until smooth. Add more water/tea for a thinner consistency.

Skin cancer develops in nearly 30% of kidney transplant recipients after about 10 years of immunosuppressants, and many times its an aggressive form.[41] Besides being careful about sun exposure, you can arm yourself with diet. Broccoli and broccoli sprouts contain a phytochemical sulforaphane, well-studied for its cancer inhibiting ability.[42] Consider this smoothie your natural sunscreen.

Nutrient Values				
	Calories	189	Potassium	607 mg
	Fat	8 g	Phosphorus	70 mg
	Fiber	8 g	Sodium	17 mg
	Protein	4 g	Calcium	61 mg

Pineapple and Beets

While we don't believe that any one food can resolve health issues, beets challenge our belief when it comes to lowering blood pressure (see below). This powerful smoothie contains a heart-healthy trifecta of nitrate, magnesium, and potassium—pressure-lowering heroes. The good fat in almonds also benefits heart health, and citrus helps you absorb the iron in beets.

- 1/2 cup 100% orange juice, calcium fortified
- 1/2 cup skim milk
- 1 cup frozen pineapple chunks, unsweetened
- 1/4 cup raw beets, peeled and diced (or use beetroot juice)
- 1/4 cup raw almond slivers

Place all ingredients into blender and mix until smooth.

Recent research published in *Hypertension* found that one cup of beetroot juice lowered blood pressure in people by 11 points within 3 to 6 hours! The effect was still present a day later.[43] The scientists explained that beets work so fast because they contain dietary nitrate, which your body converts to a gas that expands blood vessels and aids blood flow.

Nutrient Values				
	Calories	351	Potassium	926 mg
	Fat	15 g	Phosphorus	302 mg
	Fiber	7 g	Sodium	81 mg
	Protein	12 g	Calcium	265 mg

Amy's Wacky Shake

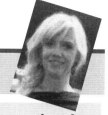

Amy knows about kidney disease since her grandmother died early from it and her mother has a transplanted kidney. Amy posted a version of this nutrient-dense smoothie on our web site at www.kidneysteps.com. Avocado in this wacky drink provides heart-healthy fats, and the fruits contain numerous antioxidants that aid in scooping up dangerous free radicals. Amy slips in a couple of powerful veggies for a high fiber content.

- 1/2 cup 100% grape juice, unsweetened
- 1/2 cup fresh spinach leaves (you won't even know it's there)
- 1/4 fresh avocado, peeled
- 1 small pear with peel, diced and cored
- 1 cup frozen blueberries, unsweetened
- 1 tsp. fresh lemon juice
- 1 T. wheat grass

Place all ingredients into blender and mix until smooth. Add a little water for a thinner consistency.

Citrus fruits (lemons, limes, oranges, grapefruit) contain naringenin, a flavonoid that successfully blocks formation of kidney cysts in the laboratory. Cysts commonly form in polycystic kidney disease (PKD), an inherited condition that usually results in dialysis. This recent discovery may lead to a treatment option.[44] Nutritious foods do contain healing substances.

Nutrient Values				
	Calories	350	Potassium	859 mg
	Fat	8 g	Phosphorus	105 mg
	Fiber	17 g	Sodium	25 mg
	Protein	5 g	Calcium	89 mg

Fig-Quinoa Breakfast

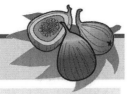

No reason to avoid breakfast with this hearty, nutritious drink. Quinoa is the "mother of all grains" with its whole-grain fiber, high-quality protein, and anti-inflammatory antioxidants. Add to that the hypertension-relieving potassium in figs, bananas, and milk, and you're set until lunch.

2 small fresh figs, diced and stem removed
1/3 cup cooked quinoa
1/2 cup skim milk
1 cup frozen banana slices (freeze in advance)
1/4 teas. ground nutmeg
1 tsp. vanilla extract

Place all ingredients into blender and mix until smooth. Add a little water for a thinner consistency.

Researchers in several studies tracked men and women for up to 20 years. Consistently, people eating breakfast most days of the week, compared to those eating breakfast 0 to 2 times a week, saw substantially reduced risks of developing diabetes, obesity, hypertension, metabolic syndrome, and abdominal fat.[45] Smoothies make breakfast easy.

Nutrient Values	Calories	324	Potassium	1,028 mg
	Fat	2 g	Phosphorus	263 mg
	Fiber	8 g	Sodium	58 mg
	Protein	9 g	Calcium	196 mg

"A" Power

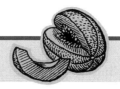

Just look at this—3 fruit servings and 2 vegetable servings in one glass. Now, that's a great start for the day. Cantaloupe, carrots, and corn supply valuable beta-carotene for vitamin A production, important in kidney disease. The potassium in the ingredients helps counter hypertension. Flax is heart- and kidney-healthy. We don't often use juice, but orange juice is associated with relieving acidosis.

1/2 cup 100% orange juice (calcium fortified)
1 cup fresh cantaloupe, diced
1/2 cup frozen corn kernels
1/2 cup frozen carrot slices
1 T. ground flax seeds
1/2 tsp. ground cinnamon

Place all ingredients into blender and mix until smooth. This is a nutrient-dense, orange-colored delight.

Yep, it's true. What's good for the heart is good for kidneys. In an analysis of 3093 participants, researchers assessed how these folks compared with the AHA's Life's Simple 7 components (see p. 9) for ideal heart health. Over the 4-year study, 160 people with CKD developed ESRD and 610 died. Those with kidney disease who had 2, 3, or 4 of the 7 components had lower rates of ESRD. Those having 5 to 7 of the components never progressed to ESRD.[46] By increasing fruit and vegetable consumption, you're on your way to slowing kidney disease progression and improving heart health.

Nutrient Values	Calories	233	Potassium	1,022 mg
	Fat	5 g	Phosphorus	160 mg
	Fiber	8 g	Sodium	74 mg
	Protein	6 g	Calcium	339 mg

Plum Pudding

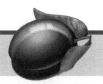

We enjoy low-fat dairy occasionally for its calcium and heart-health benefits. This high potassium shake also helps offset over-consumption of sodium for improved blood pressure control. Plums are shown to lower diabetes risk.

1 cup skim milk
2 ripe plums, pitted and diced
1 cup banana slices, frozen
1/4 tsp. ground cinnamon
1/4 cup oat flakes (we use old fashioned oats)

Place all ingredients in blender and mix until smooth. Add some crushed ice if you want a slushier drink.

Kidney patients have an elevated risk for strokes, as well as related cardiovascular events. In a large population-based study, Swedish researchers found that the greater the consumption of low-fat dairy (milk, yogurt), the lower the risk of suffering a stroke.[47]

Nutrient Values				
	Calories	358	Potassium	1,205 mg
	Fat	2 g	Phosphorus	385 mg
	Fiber	8 g	Sodium	106 mg
	Protein	14 g	Calcium	339 mg

Pom Power

Pomegranate juice, with its powerful antioxidants, offers several benefits to kidney patients. Pom's ascorbic acid and polyphenolic flavonoids may help kidney patients improve lipid and cholesterol levels, thereby decreasing risk for cardiovascular disease. Pom also promotes detoxification and may inhibit come cancers.

Individuals taking cyclosporin or tacrolimus should substitute a different liquid for pomegranate. Pom can interfere with absorption of those immuno-suppressants.

1/2 cup 100% pomegranate juice, unsweetened
1/2 cup water
1/2 single-serve container nonfat, plain Greek yogurt
1 cup frozen pineapple chunks, unsweetened
1/4 cup oat flakes
1/2 tsp. ground cinnamon

Place all ingredients into blender and mix until smooth for a delicious treat.

Pomegranate and its juice do more than just look succulent. Pomegranate contains powerful antioxidants that serve as natural antibacterials and antivirals. Pom is shown to protect beneficial intestinal microbes; reduce inflammation of gums; inhibit antibiotic-resistant bacteria; and, lower risks for viral infections such as the flu, colds, and sinus infections.[18]

Nutrient Values				
	Calories	279	Potassium	645 mg
	Fat	2 g	Phosphorus	226 mg
	Fiber	5 g	Sodium	45 mg
	Protein	12 g	Calcium	153 mg

Diabetes Relief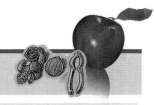

We specifically chose the three fruits in this smoothie because they were the top three fruits in the study below for lowering diabetes risk. We added heart-healthy nuts and whole-grain quinoa because they also may lower diabetes risk and protect the cardiovascular system. Besides offering real nutrition, this baby is tasty!

3/4 cup water
1/2 medium apple with peel, cored and chopped
1/2 cup frozen blueberries, unsweetened
1/2 cup (about 15) red seedless grapes, frozen
1/4 cup cooked quinoa
1/4 cup raw walnuts
1/2 tsp. ground cinnamon

Place water and apple into blender and mix until smooth. Add remaining ingredients, blending well. We sometimes substitute blackberries for blueberries.

Whole fruit is not a diabetic's enemy, but juice may be. In fact, eating more fruit offers diabetes protection, while drinking fruit juice raises diabetes risk. In a study of nearly 200,000 health professionals, substituting just 3 servings of whole fruit for juice per week was associated with significantly lowered odds of type 2 diabetes (and, therefore, CKD). The advantage was greatest with blueberries at 26% lowered odds with 3 weekly servings. Apples and grapes also ranked high.[49]

Nutrient Values				
	Calories	389	Potassium	504 mg
	Fat	20 g	Phosphorus	206 mg
	Fiber	10 g	Sodium	9 mg
	Protein	8 g	Calcium	75 mg

Blackberry Sun Shield

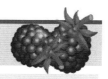

Blackberries top the list of foods highest in antioxidant phytochemicals. Their health-promoting compounds—ellagic acid, quercetin, and several anthocyanins—inhibit some cancer tumors. Anthocyanins may serve as a natural sunscreen, particularly important to kidney patients, including transplant recipients.

1 cup 100% coconut water, unsweetened
1 cup frozen blackberries, unsweetened
1/2 cup banana, sliced
1 tsp. fresh ginger, chopped
2 T. wheat germ

Place all ingredients into your blender, and mix until smooth. If you prefer gluten-free, substitute ground flaxseed or nuts for the wheat germ.

Kidney patients, including transplant recipients, have higher rates of skin and other cancers than seen in the general population. Cancer rate in CKD is estimated to be about 20% higher than normal. Anthocyanins in this smoothie inhibit oxidative stress caused by the sun and arm us against several other common cancers.[50]

Nutrient Values				
	Calories	264	Potassium	1,215 mg
	Fat	3 g	Phosphorus	231 mg
	Fiber	14 g	Sodium	258 mg
	Protein	8 g	Calcium	112 mg

Eva's Pink Shake

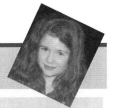

Eight-year-old Eva loves pink, even in her smoothies. Eva probably isn't aware that the ingredients in this delicious mix rank high in reducing acidosis, a state common in kidney patients. Fruit and veggies contain phytochemicals that help counter hypertension and internal inflammation, also common in kidney disease. So far, Eva shows no signs of Alport Syndrome, the inherited kidney disease plaguing many in her family.

1/2 cup almond milk, unsweetened (we use Silk brand)
1/4 cup water
1/2 cup banana slices, frozen
1/2 single-serving container nonfat, plain Greek yogurt (3 ounces)
1/4 cup fresh or frozen carrots, sliced
1/4 cup frozen corn kernels
1/2 cup frozen raspberries, unsweetened

Place all ingredients into blender and mix until smooth. Add more liquid for a thinner consistency.

Acidosis is prevalent among CKD patients, including kidney transplant recipients. Poor diet and immunosuppressants contribute to acidosis. Researchers looked at diets of transplant recipients. Compared to recipients consuming higher amounts of fruits and vegetables, those with higher intakes of animal protein (from meat, cheese, and fish) registered greater levels of acidosis.[51]

Nutrient Values				
	Calories	206	Potassium	646 mg
	Fat	3 g	Phosphorus	194 mg
	Fiber	8 g	Sodium	131 mg
	Protein	12 g	Calcium	352 mg

Pear-Hemp Shake

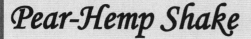

Hemp is often called the most complete food in the world, a tall claim. However, hemp is exceptionally rich in plant protein, omega fatty acids, and most vitamins and minerals. Pears are a good source of fiber and have glutathione, an antioxidant tied to reducing risk of hypertension, stroke, and cancer.

1/2 cup coconut water
1/2 cup frozen raspberries, unsweetened
1 medium pear with peel, diced and cored
3 T. hemp seeds
2 fresh mint leaves

Place all ingredients into blender and mix until smooth.

Fruits and vegetables (F+V) work well to relieve acidosis. Scientists divided stage 4 kidney patients into 3 groups. One group received extra F+V; the second group received sodium bicarbonate pills; the third group received neither. After a year, GFR and kidney function had worsened in the third group. The F+V and the bicarbonate groups had improved metabolic acidosis and similar preservation of kidney function. The extra F+V did NOT cause hyperkalemia (high potassium), either.[52]

Nutrient Values				
	Calories	281	Potassium	497 mg
	Fat	15 g	Phosphorus	433 mg
	Fiber	9 g	Sodium	128 mg
	Protein	13 g	Calcium	53 mg

Part 5
Smoothies with Reduced Phosphorus and Potassium

Your renal dietitian or nephrologist will let you know if your blood tests indicate you must reduce your dietary intake of foods high in phosphorus and potassium. A rise in blood serum phosphorus above 4.6 mg/dL or potassium above 5.0 mg/dL means your deteriorating kidneys are unable to keep blood levels of these minerals stable.

You obtain phosphorus and potassium from your diet, and both nutrients are critical to good health. However, consuming foods high in these minerals becomes dangerous to your cardiovascular system and your remaining kidney function when your kidneys can no longer balance amounts retained in your blood. If blood levels are consistently high, the kidney patient can suffer heart attack, heart failure, or stroke.

Most kidney patients who must lower dietary intake of these nutrients are limited to about 1000 mg/day of phosphorus (your body only needs 700 mg/day) and 2,000 to 3,000 mg/day of potassium (the RDA for an adult is 4700 mg/day). However, your renal dietitian will instruct you as to your specific limits, if that time comes.

The smoothies in Part 5 provide well under one-third of those maximum limits, leaving plenty of room for inclusion of additional healthy foods in your remaining daily meals and snacks. Several smoothies in the previous Part 4 also fall under the "1/3 of your maximum limit" for phosphorus and potassium. So, you can enjoy those, too.

All the smoothies in Part 6 (for dialysis) are appropriate for you, so long as you keep an eye on your total grams of protein for the day. While a kidney patient should limit protein to modest levels before dialysis, the dialysis patient must increase protein.

You will want to provide all smoothie recipes you intend to try to your renal dietitian to assure they are appropriate in view of your specific blood test results.

Touch of Green

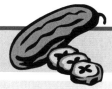

High cholesterol is more common in kidney patients than in the general population. Kidney patients also suffer from destructive metabolic acidosis and inflammation. The ingredients of this pale-colored smoothie just might help lessen these conditions.

- 1/2 cup freshly brewed green tea, cooled
- 1/2 cup frozen pineapple, unsweetened
- 1/4 cup cucumber with peel, diced
- 1/4 cup celery, chopped
- 1/2 tsp. ground cinnamon
- 1 T. ground flax seeds

Place all ingredients in blender and mix until smooth.

Is cinnamon a statin substitute? Statins are overprescribed to kidney patients, says recent research.[1] Cinnamon is not. Diabetic patients given varying amounts of cinnamon for 4 to 18 weeks saw statistically significant reductions in fasting blood glucose and total cholesterol; decreases in bad triglycerides and LDLs; and increases in good HDL cholesterol.[2] Now, you know why we put cinnamon in so many smoothies.

Nutrient Values	Calories	90	Potassium	271 mg
	Fat	3 g	Phosphorus	66 mg
	Fiber	4 g	Sodium	26 mg
	Protein	2 g	Calcium	58 mg

Nausea Buster

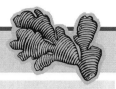

Ginger's antioxidant gingerol shows anti-inflammatory, pain-relieving properties that act as a digestive tonic. Blueberries contain anthocyanins that help the body eliminate toxins. Pineapple and mint are known digestive aids. Sip this little snack to ease a tummy upset.

1/2 cup water or freshly brewed green tea, cooled
1/2 cup frozen pineapple chunks, unsweetened
1/2 cup frozen blueberries, unsweetened
2 tsp. fresh ginger root, chopped
2 large or 4 small peppermint leaves, fresh

Place all ingredients in blender and blend until smooth, adding more liquid as needed. We prefer green tea in this recipe because of its warming and antimicrobial effect.

Later stages of CKD often are accompanied by nausea resulting from a build up of toxins that malfunctioning kidneys fail to filter from the blood. Ginger is shown to possess free radical-scavenging, antioxidant, and lipid-improving properties, which may be tied to its gastro-protective abilities.[3]

Nutrient Values				
	Calories	85	Potassium	156 mg
	Fat	0 g	Phosphorus	19 mg
	Fiber	4 g	Sodium	4 mg
	Protein	1 g	Calcium	24 mg

Berries for Pressure Relief

Reduced blood pressure is a goal of this beauty. Dark berries are known for their anthocyanins, antioxidants that may lower blood pressure and decrease arterial stiffness for cardiovascular protection. Flax contains heart-healthy fats and additional fiber, both heart protective.

1 cup unsweetened almond milk (we use Silk brand)
1/2 cup fresh or frozen strawberries, unsweetened
1/2 cup frozen blueberries, unsweetened
1/2 cup frozen blackberries, unsweetened
1 T. ground flax seeds

Place all ingredients in blender and mix until smooth. Using mostly frozen berries provides a lusciously thick texture. Kids love this smoothie.

Kidney patients are 23 times (yikes!) more likely to develop cardiovascular disease; and for them, it's the leading cause of death.[4] Diet changes those odds. In a study of 1,898 women, researchers found that the highest average intakes of anthocyanins were associated with lower blood pressure and arterial pressure (pressure of circulating blood in arteries). Researchers concluded that 1 to 2 berry servings a day may be enough.[5] This smoothie provides 3 berry servings.

Nutrient Values				
	Calories	162	Potassium	356 mg
	Fat	6 g	Phosphorus	107 mg
	Fiber	11 g	Sodium	157 mg
	Protein	4 g	Calcium	514 mg

Jennifer's Drinkable Pumpkin Pie

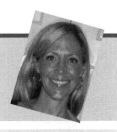

Yes, pumpkin is relatively high in potassium, but the small amount in this smoothie, along with the mango, offers you the benefits of beta-carotene and vitamin A. Beta-carotene gives vegetables and fruits their orange color and is an antioxidant that may slow the oxidative stress that contributes to progression of kidney disease. Dietary sources, rather than pills, are safe.

- 1/2 cup unsweetened almond milk
- 1/2 cup water
- 1/4 cup 100% pumpkin puree, unsweetened
- 1/2 cup frozen mango chunks, unsweetened
- 1/4 cup oat flakes (we use old-fashioned oat flakes)
- 1/2 tsp. ground pumpkin pie spice mix

Place all ingredients in blender and mix until smooth.

Obesity is epidemic in the U.S. and is now a recognized cause of kidney disease, termed "obesity-related glomerulopathy." Obesity also impacts the outcomes of other kidney diseases, causing faster progression of kidney damage and a doubling of the likelihood of reaching end stage.[6] Low-cal smoothies like this one help you lose weight.

Nutrient Values				
	Calories	166	Potassium	362 mg
	Fat	3 g	Phosphorus	127 mg
	Fiber	6 g	Sodium	80 mg
	Protein	5 g	Calcium	267 mg

Vitamin C Delight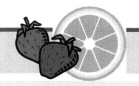

This smoothie-snack provides 100% of your daily vitamin C requirement, which kidney patients want, but not much more. Too much vitamin C or not enough can be kidney-harmful. A powerful antioxidant and immunity modulator, vitamin C helps bind nasty free radicals, reducing risk of illness.

1/2 cup water
1/2 cup fresh navel orange segments
1/2 cup frozen strawberries, unsweetened
1 T. fresh parsley, chopped
1 T. ground flax seeds

Place all ingredients in blender and mix until smooth.

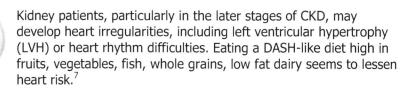

Kidney patients, particularly in the later stages of CKD, may develop heart irregularities, including left ventricular hypertrophy (LVH) or heart rhythm difficulties. Eating a DASH-like diet high in fruits, vegetables, fish, whole grains, low fat dairy seems to lessen heart risk.[7]

Nutrient Values				
	Calories	67	Potassium	326 mg
	Fat	3 g	Phosphorus	76 mg
	Fiber	6 g	Sodium	7 mg
	Protein	3 g	Calcium	71 mg

Swigging Salad

This strange-colored but tasty smoothie provides over two servings of vegetables with their health-promoting antioxidants, as well as the omega-3 fatty acids in olive oil and sunflower seeds. Omega-3s are cardio-protective, associated with reduced triglycerides, inflammation, and oxidative stress. Garlic aids heart health by slowing plaque progression in blood vessels.

1/2 cup water
2 tsp. extra virgin olive oil
1 tsp. fresh lemon juice
1/4 cup fresh cucumber (with peel), chopped
1/4 cup fresh red pepper, diced
2 cherry tomatoes
1/2 glove fresh garlic, chopped
1 medium radish, chopped
1 fresh sage leaf
1 T. raw sunflower seeds
1 cup fresh red leaf lettuce, chopped

Place all ingredients except the lettuce in blender, mix until smooth. Add the lettuce, and blend to desired consistency. Sprinkle in some freshly ground black pepper. Reduce the water and add 1/2 cup crushed ice for a colder, thicker drink.

Research suggests that garlic acts like an ACE inhibitor to relax blood vessels. In three trials, researchers also found that damaging plaque progression in blood vessels slowed by 50% in those taking garlic extract.[8] The actual garlic in this smoothie is better.

Nutrient Values				
	Calories	161	Potassium	330 mg
	Fat	14 g	Phosphorus	94 mg
	Fiber	3 g	Sodium	15 mg
	Protein	3 g	Calcium	31 mg

Going Chinese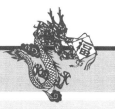

This low-cal drink packs a nutritional cancer-fighting punch. Cabbage contains sulforaphane, found to activate enzymes that defend against carcinogens— important to kidney patients, who develop cancer at higher rates than the general population.

1/4 cup water or freshly brewed green tea, cooled
1/2 tsp. fresh ginger root, chopped
1/4 cup celery, chopped
1 T. fresh chives, chopped
1/2 cup bok choy (Chinese cabbage), chopped
1/4 cup bean sprouts
1/4 cup fresh red sweet pepper, diced
1/2 tsp. sesame oil
1 tsp. sesame seeds
1/2 cup crushed ice

Place all ingredients in blender and mix until smooth. You may need to add a tablespoon of additional water for blending. Sprinkle with freshly ground black pepper.

Up to 35% of cancers are diet-related, resulting from nitrates and nitrites in processed meats; high consumption of red meat; charcoal cooking; and over-consumption of trans fats, saturated fats, and sugar.[9] A recent study found a significantly decreased risk of renal cancer in people with the highest consumption of cruciferous vegetables.[10] Regulary enjoy cabbage, broccoli, Brussels sprouts, and cauliflower.

Nutrient Values				
	Calories	69	Potassium	301 mg
	Fat	4 g	Phosphorus	63 mg
	Fiber	3 g	Sodium	26 mg
	Protein	3 g	Calcium	77 mg

Snack for Lower BP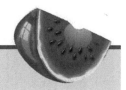

This little red jewel can satisfy that afternoon desire for a sweet snack while doing your body good. In studies, watermelon lowered blood pressure, and antioxidants in the red grapes and mint helped counter disease-causing inflammation.

1 cup watermelon, diced
1/2 cup red grapes (about 15), frozen in advance
2 fresh mint leaves
1/4 cup water
1/2 cup crushed ice

Place all ingredients in blender and mix until smooth.

Don't drink red wine? Red grapes may be the next best thing when it comes to health benefits. Numerous studies evidence that phytochemicals in grapes have anticancer effects and help lower risk for cardiovascular disease.[11] Kidney patients, even with early kidney deterioration, have substantially increased risks for heart and blood vessel issues. Smoothies like this are heart-protective.

Nutrient Values			
Calories	98	Potassium	315 mg
Fat	0 g	Phosphorus	32 mg
Fiber	2 g	Sodium	4 mg
Protein	2 g	Calcium	20 mg

Diabetes Ammunition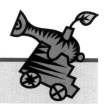

Fruits are rich in health-promoting antioxidants and phytochemicals, and fruit consumption is linked to prevention of many chronic diseases, including heart disease, kidney disease, and diabetes. For diabetes prevention, the fruits selected for this smoothie may be better than others.

1/2 cup water
1/2 cup frozen blueberries, unsweetened
1/2 cup apple with peel, diced
1/2 cup grapes, frozen in advance
1 T. unsalted peanut butter (only ingredient is peanuts)

Place all ingredients in blender and mix until smooth. This thick smoothie has a distinct peanut butter taste.

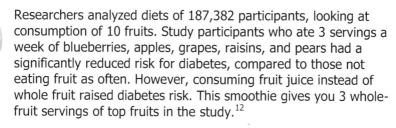

Researchers analyzed diets of 187,382 participants, looking at consumption of 10 fruits. Study participants who ate 3 servings a week of blueberries, apples, grapes, raisins, and pears had a significantly reduced risk for diabetes, compared to those not eating fruit as often. However, consuming fruit juice instead of whole fruit raised diabetes risk. This smoothie gives you 3 whole-fruit servings of top fruits in the study.[12]

Nutrient Values	Calories	218	Potassium	363 mg
	Fat	8 g	Phosphorus	88 mg
	Fiber	6 g	Sodium	8 mg
	Protein	5 g	Calcium	31 mg

Tropical Delight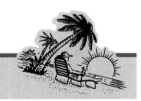

Life is good with the sweet taste of tropical fruits packed with vitamin C and disease-fighting antioxidants. Sneaking in a vegetable makes this smoothie even better. Green, leafy lettuces are alkaline-inducing, helping to lower damaging blood acidosis common in kidney disease. Cinnamon helps control blood pressure, and the almond milk supplies loads of calcium.

1 cup unsweetened almond milk (we use Silk brand)
1/2 cup frozen pineapple chunks, unsweetened
1/2 cup frozen mango cubes, unsweetened
1/2 cup fresh red leaf lettuce, chopped
1/4 tsp. ground cinnamon

Place all ingredients in blender and mix until smooth. Add 1/4 cup of water for a thinner consistency.

Increased uric acid levels commonly occur in kidney patients as failing kidneys lose the ability to filter the toxin from the blood. Uric acid is associated with elevated blood pressure, metabolic syndrome, acidosis, and progression of kidney disease. Reduce uric acid levels by cutting sugar and high fructose corn syrup from your diet.[13]

Nutrient Values				
	Calories	326	Potassium	296 mg
	Fat	3 g	Phosphorus	45 mg
	Fiber	4 g	Sodium	156 mg
	Protein	2 g	Calcium	488 mg

Live Long and Prosper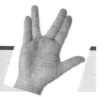

Consuming wholesome foods allows you to enjoy a longer life, even in kidney disease. Fruits and vegetables are fountains of youth with disease-fighting antioxidants. The vitamin C stars of this smoothie work to resist infections, help to lower blood pressure and heart disease risk, and aid in absorption of iron. Basil may help prevent free radical damage that causes disease and aging.

1/2 cup water or freshly brewed green tea, cooled
1/2 cup navel orange, peeled and sectioned
1 tsp. fresh orange zest
1/3 cup Nasoya extra-firm tofu (you'll never know it's there)
2 fresh basil leaves
1/2 cup frozen raspberries, unsweetened

Place all ingredients in blender, adding the raspberries last. Mix until smooth. If the smoothie is a little too tart, add a teaspoon of honey for an additional 4 mg. of potassium.

Current reviews indicate that antioxidants help prevent progression of kidney disease to end stage, lower creatinine levels, improve creatinine clearance, and lessen oxidative stress in kidney patients.[14] Good reasons to get your fruits and vegetables.

Nutrient Values				
	Calories	149	Potassium	233 mg
	Fat	5 g	Phosphorus	108 mg
	Fiber	7 g	Sodium	5 mg
	Protein	10 g	Calcium	113 mg

UTI and Stone Defense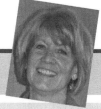

I love this smoothie. Cranberries are high in important disease-fighting antioxidants and anti-inflammatories, as are blueberries, ginger, and cinnamon. Blueberries and oats help cut risks of heart attacks and memory loss, say researchers.

1/2 cup 100% cranberry juice, unsweetened
1/2 cup water
1 cup frozen blueberries, unsweetened
1/4 cup oat flakes (we use old-fashioned oats straight from container)
1 tsp. fresh ginger root, chopped
1/2 tsp. ground cinnamon

Place all ingredients in blender and blend until smooth. This smoothie is a little tart. If it is too tart for you, add honey (4 mg. potassium/tsp) or maple syrup (14 mg. potassium/tsp).

A 2013 study of 240,000 adults found that 20,000 of them experienced kidney stones. In a 24-year follow-up, women with stones were 30% more likely to develop heart disease.[15] What to do? Limit salt and meat/egg protein; drink plenty of fluids (including cranberry juice) if you are not fluid-limited; and eat loads of fruits and vegetables not otherwise restricted because of your type of stone.

Nutrient Values				
	Calories	220	Potassium	279 mg
	Fat	2 g	Phosphorus	119 mg
	Fiber	9 g	Sodium	8 mg
	Protein	4 g	Calcium	58 mg

Taste of Turmeric

Turmeric is linked to many health benefits. The curcumin in turmeric might protect against advancing kidney disease, cardiovascular disease, high cholesterol, stomach issues, and cancer. You obtain turmeric's full benefits when it is paired with a little fat (in the ricotta cheese). The nutritious berries are an antioxidant bonus.

1/2 cup frozen blackberries, unsweetened
1/2 cup frozen strawberries, unsweetened
1/4 cup low fat ricotta cheese
1/2 tsp. fresh ginger root, chopped or grated
1/4 tsp. ground turmeric
3/4 cup water or freshly brewed green tea, cooled

Place all ingredients in blender and blend until smooth. If this smoothie is not sweet enough for you, add a teaspoon of honey for 4 mg. of potassium.

Scientists are feverishly researching the benefits of turmeric and its component curcumin. Turmeric may have far-reaching benefits in CKD. It appears to preserve kidney function, protect transplanted kidneys, preserve heart and cell health in kidney disease; and its antioxidants decrease oxidative stress in CKD.[16] Will turmeric prove to be a kidney patient's dream spice?

Nutrient Values	Calories	138	Potassium	314 mg
	Fat	5 g	Phosphorus	149 mg
	Fiber	6 g	Sodium	64 mg
	Protein	8 g	Calcium	204 mg

Fitting in a Power Vege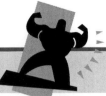

This light snack is heavy on nutrients. Spinach, lauded as a vegetable superstar, may decrease risks for heart disease and cancer, says research. Papaya contains carpain, a calming chemical. Pineapple's bromelin may help relieve arthritis. For better health, down this smoothie rather than grabbing a soft drink.

1/2 cup fresh papaya, peeled and diced
1/2 cup frozen pineapple chunks, unsweetened
1/2 cup unsweetened almond milk (we use Silk brand)
1/2 cup fresh spinach
1 T. hemp seeds
1/2 tsp. ground cinnamon

Place all ingredients in blender and blend until smooth. Add a little water if you want a thinner consistency.

 Sure, drinking sweetened colas substantially increases risk for CKD. Diet sodas are bad, too. An examination of 24 studies on artificially sweetened beverages revealed these drinks substantially increased risks for metabolic syndrome, diabetes, hypertension, and coronary heart disease.[17] Prior studies evidenced that drinking more than one diet soda a day significantly increased albuminuria and speeded kidney function decline by as much as 30%.[18]

Nutrient Values				
	Calories	148	Potassium	326 mg
	Fat	7 g	Phosphorus	32 mg
	Fiber	4 g	Sodium	94 mg
	Protein	6 g	Calcium	268 mg

Soy and Sage Power

Sage is rich in antioxidants and vitamin K and may help relieve agitation and improve memory, says research. Sage, along with antioxidant-rich blueberries and pears, helps counter harmful systemic inflammation characteristic in kidney disease. Soy (tofu) provides kidney-kind vegetable protein.

1/2 cup water or freshly brewed green tea, cooled
1/2 cup fresh pear with peel, diced
1 cup frozen blueberries, unsweetened
1/2 cup extra firm tofu, Nasoya brand
1 T. fresh sage, chopped

Place all ingredients in blender and mix until smooth.

Unfolding research indicates that soy (from fermented beans) beats meat as a protein choice for kidney patients. Unlike meat sources, vegetable sources of protein help keep phosphorus levels in check.[19] Soy may also lower cholesterol, and its isoflavones and phytoestrogens may have beneficial effects on osteoporosis and cardiovascular disease.[20]

Nutrient Values				
	Calories	209	Potassium	209 mg
	Fat	4 g	Phosphorus	100 mg
	Fiber	11 g	Sodium	25 mg
	Protein	9 g	Calcium	125 mg

Part 6
Smoothies for Dialysis

Dialysis presents numerous dietary challenges because it can only replace one aspect of kidney function–the removal of waste and fluids accumulating in the body between dialysis sessions. The waste and fluids come from foods and beverages you consume and the natural and necessary metabolism of these substances by your body's cells to create energy for living.

Unlike working kidneys, dialysis cannot balance certain chemicals obtained from food. Dialysis is also unable to trigger the manufacture of red blood cells to avoid anemia; convert vitamin D obtained from sunlight and foods into the form the body can use; or stimulate use of calcium for bone health. These missing kidney functions must be accommodated by dietary restrictions and medications.

Often, dialysis patients are told to limit fluid to a liter or so a day; to increase protein and calorie intake to avoid muscle wasting and malnutrition; to increase sodium intake to replace sodium lost in dialysis; and, to limit dietary intake of potassium, phosphorus and, perhaps, calcium. These restrictions make diet selections difficult, particularly in the beginning, and require careful focus and planning to maintain good nutrition.

Involvement of a renal dietitian is vital in structuring an appropriate and nutritious eating plan. The type of dialysis you choose and how often you dialyze will partially determine what and how much you can eat and drink. Likewise, your age, weight, and other health issues (such as diabetes, heart disease) will impact your particular renal diet.

The following smoothies are renal dietitian reviewed and approved and can be a nutritious part of your renal diet. They may serve as a pleasant and fun change from your regular food choices. You and your dietitian will want to examine the nutritional content provided for each smoothie to assure it fits within your individualized version of a renal diet.

You may enjoy many of the smoothies in Part 5, as well. They are also lower in potassium and phosphorus. Be sure to include the fluid in the smoothies toward your total fluid intake for the day, if you are fluid-restricted.

Blueberry Starter

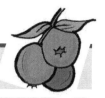

We like this antioxidant starter in the morning for a day of free-radical fighting, heart protection, and blood pressure control. Blueberries are antioxidant superstars with their protective anthocyanins. Oats guard cardiovascular health, and yogurt may help lower blood pressure, say researchers.

1 cup frozen blueberries, unsweetened
1/2 single-serving container nonfat, plain Greek yogurt (3 ounces)
1/4 cup oat flakes (we use old-fashioned oats)
1/4 tsp. ground nutmeg
1/2 cup water

Place all ingredients into blender and mix until smooth. Use less water for a thicker smoothie.

A recent survey reports that most dialysis patients do a poor job of restricting dietary phosphorus intake, and it appears linked to consumption of fast foods and fizzy drinks that contain lots of hidden phosphates.[1] Smoothies are a better "fast food," and you can easily keep track of, and control, the phosphorus content. Why not forego McDonald's and those nutritionally worthless colas?

Nutrient Values				
	Calories	210	Potassium	290 mg
	Fat	2 g	Phosphorus	217 mg
	Fiber	7 g	Sodium	36 mg
	Protein	12 g	Calcium	130 mg

Berry-Orange Inflammation Fighter

The wonderfully delicious combination of raspberries and orange is a rich source of health-benefiting phytochemicals and vitamin C, protective against infections, inflammation, and cancer. The antioxidants in these fruits scavenge harmful free radicals to reduce disease state. Cottage cheese, a low fat dairy, provides some vitamin D.

1/2 cup water or freshly brewed green tea, cooled
1/2 cup frozen raspberries, unsweetened
1/2 cup navel orange sections
1 tsp. fresh orange zest
1/2 cup 1% low fat cottage cheese (we used "no-sodium," you may need the sodium)
1/2 tsp. ground cinnamon

Place all ingredients into blender and mix until smooth.

In a sample of 256 dialysis patients, 151 had diabetes and were more likely to be vitamin D deficient. They also had a higher prevalence of coronary artery disease and obesity. However, those treated with vitamin D2 (rather than vitamin D3) showed a significant reduction in risk of vascular access problems during dialysis.[2] Ask your doctor about D2.

Nutrient Values	Calories	158	Potassium	337 mg
	Fat	2 g	Phosphorus	189 mg
	Fiber	7 g	Sodium	17 mg
	Protein	16 g	Calcium	135 mg

Blueberry Cheesecake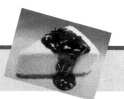

By now, you know how much we admire those little deep-blue pearls of antioxidants called blueberries. They zero in on many kidney-disease issues, including chronic inflammation, hypertension, acidosis. Blueberries and flax are loaded with fiber for cardiovascular protection. This is one of our favorite combinations of the two.

1/2 cup unsweetened almond milk
1 cup frozen blueberries
1/2 tsp. ground nutmeg
1/4 cup ricotta cheese, part skim milk
1 T. ground flax seeds

Place all ingredients into blender and mix until smooth.

Chronic inflammation is a disease-promoting state common in CKD, including in dialysis. It is associated with a decreased survival prognosis. Researchers divided dialysis patients into two groups. One group received flaxseed oil for 120 days and the other received mineral oil. One-third of the flax group moved from "inflamed" to "non-inflamed," compared to only 16% of the mineral oil group.[3] Enjoy flax for increased survival.

Nutrient Values				
	Calories	220	Potassium	250 mg
	Fat	10 g	Phosphorus	187 mg
	Fiber	9 g	Sodium	142 mg
	Protein	10 g	Calcium	437 mg

Heart Blush

This tart, pale pink goodie aims straight for heart protection. Pomegranate is chock full of newfound benefits for dialysis patients. It can improve blood pressure and lower risk to cardiovascular health. Likewise, low fat dairy and basil are shown to have positive effects on blood pressure and heart health.

1/4 cup 100% pomegranate juice, unsweetened
1/2 cup frozen pineapple chunks, unsweetened
2 fresh basil leaves
1/2 single-serving container nonfat, plain Greek yogurt (3 ounces)

Place all ingredients into blender and mix until smooth. Add a tablespoon or two of water if needed for blending.

In a study of 101 hemodialysis patients, half received 100cc (about 1/2 cup) of pomegranate juice 3 times/week for one year, and half received a placebo. The pomegranate group saw declines in oxidative stress, blood pressure, lipid and cholesterol levels, and metabolic inflammation—real benefits for heart health. In the placebo group, 50% worsened in these areas.[4] Pomegranate is high in potassium, a problem for many dialysis patients. Its multiple heart health benefits, though, make it worth incorporating into your diet after discussion with your dietitian.

Nutrient Values	Calories	125	Potassium	346 mg
	Fat	1 g	Phosphorus	131 mg
	Fiber	2 g	Sodium	38 mg
	Protein	9 g	Calcium	114 mg

Red Velvet Chocolate Delight

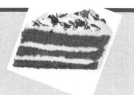

Cocoa, the star of this smoothie, is shown to promote cardiovascular health, lower bad LDL's, raise good HDL's, and cut cancer risk. Cocoa also acts as a mood lifter by stimulating release of endorphins in the brain. The fruit offers additional antioxidants to promote better health.

1/2 cup frozen raspberries, unsweetened
1/2 cup frozen pineapple chunks, unsweetened
1 tsp. dark cocoa powder, unsweetened
1 cup almond milk, unsweetened (we use Silk brand)
1 scoop vanilla whey powder (we use Biochem)

Place all ingredients into blender and mix until smooth.

Obesity helps drive CKD to end stage and dialysis. Polyphenols and flavanols in cocoa may aid in reducing body weight. Researchers are exploring just why cocoa reduces the digestion and absorption of fats and carbohydrates.[5] A little cocoa goes a long way, given that most people consume it as sweetened, fatty concoctions. This smoothie uses the more healthful unsweetened cocoa powder.

Nutrient Values				
	Calories	162	Potassium	289 mg
	Fat	3 g	Phosphorus	84 mg
	Fiber	7 g	Sodium	174 mg
	Protein	13 g	Calcium	526 mg

Blueberry-Peach Tummy Soother

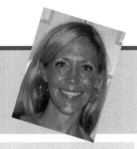

Rosemary has a long reputation for calming nerves and enhancing memory. It is used here for its antiseptic, antiviral, and anti-inflammatory features. Ginger is known to relieve nausea.[6] I can't resist the blueberries and peaches for their kidney-friendly, anti-inflammatory effects.

1/2 cup water or freshly brewed green tea, cooled
1/2 cup frozen blueberries, unsweetened
1/2 cup fresh peach slices
1/4 cup oat flakes (we use old-fashioned oats)
3/4 tsp. fresh ginger root, chopped
1/2 tsp fresh rosemary leaves, finely chopped
1 scoop whey protein powder (we use Biochem)

Place all ingredients into blender and mix until smooth. We sometimes omit the whey powder for an even more delightful flavor.

Restless legs syndrome (RLS) is a common dialysis concern. In a study of 24 dialysis patients with RLS, those who used an exercise bike for 45 minutes/3 times a week, adding resistance (making pedaling harder) over time, saw a 58% decline in RLS symptoms after six months, compared to non-resistance pedalers.[7] Researchers noted that improvement in cardio ability was the key.

Nutrient Values				
Calories	203	Potassium	319 mg
Fat	2 g	Phosphorus	133 mg
Fiber	6 g	Sodium	24 mg
Protein	14 g	Calcium	77 mg

Rice Pudding

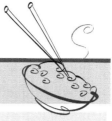

A date is like candy—sticky and delicious. While the white rice is not as nutritious as brown, this processed version contains much less potassium and retains important protein and B vitamins. Also, the drink is loaded with calcium.

1/2 cup unsweetened vanilla almond milk
   (we use Silk brand)
1/2 cup cooked white rice
1/4 cup ricotta cheese, part skim milk
1/2 tsp. cinnamon
1 Madjool date, diced finely
1 tsp. honey

Place all ingredients into a high-powered blender and mix until smooth. For a slushier texture, add 1/2 cup crushed ice.

You may avoid nuts because of their high phosphorus/potassium content. Almond milk has little of both minerals but provides some of the amazing benefits of whole nuts. In a recent study involving 120,000 men and women, daily nut eaters decreased their risk of early death from kidney and other diseases by 20%, compared to an only 7% decrease in those having nuts just once a week.[8]

Nutrient Values	Calories	294	Potassium	301 mg
	Fat	6 g	Phosphorus	173 mg
	Fiber	3 g	Sodium	137 mg
	Protein	10 g	Calcium	430 mg

Pear-Seeds-Pineapple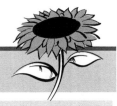

Turmeric is studied for its cancer-fighting tendencies. It also aids the liver in detoxification and may help to relieve side effects of chemotherapy. Pears and pineapple assist in reducing disease-causing inflammation. Sunflower seeds provide heart-healthy fats.

1/2 cup fresh pear with peel, diced
1/2 cup frozen pineapple chunks, unsweetened
1/2 single-serving container nonfat, plain Greek yogurt (3 ounces)
1/4 tsp. ground turmeric
1 T. raw sunflower seeds
1/2 cup water or freshly brewed green tea, cooled

Place all ingredients into blender and mix until smooth.

 Always sleepy? You're not alone. In a survey of dialysis patients, up to 80% reported sleep apnea, a disruption in breathing during sleep. Sleep apnea is associated with hypertension. About 70% of patients reported excessive daytime sleepiness; 41% unwillingly fell asleep during the day; and 31% reported decreased concentration.[9] Speak with your doctor about sleep issues. They can be relieved.

Nutrient Values	Calories	190	Potassium	376 mg
	Fat	5 g	Phosphorus	193 mg
	Fiber	5 g	Sodium	34 mg
	Protein	11 g	Calcium	120 mg

Touch of Fig

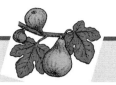

This thick smoothie allows you to enjoy the health benefits of the fig. Figs are naturally rich in phytochemicals, antioxidants, and vitamins. Chlorogince in figs seems to aid in regulating blood sugar levels in diabetes. Figs' iron is helpful in CKD, too.

1/2 cup crushed ice
1 fresh small fig, diced
10 red grapes, frozen in advance
1/4 cup ricotta cheese, part-skim milk
1/2 tsp. vanilla extract
1/4 tsp. ground cinnamon

Place all ingredients into blender and mix until smooth. You may wish to add a little water for a thinner consistency.

Researchers recently looked at outcomes for dialysis patients seen by nephrologists taking care of 50 to 200 patients. Patient survival was better when the nephrologist had around 65 or fewer patients. Nephrologists with smaller caseloads saw patients more frequently and for longer periods. Patients had higher transplant rates, higher Kt/Vs, and longer durations of treatment. Ask your doc how many patients he/she sees. [10]

Nutrient Values				
	Calories	159	Potassium	270 mg
	Fat	5 g	Phosphorus	127 mg
	Fiber	2 g	Sodium	62 mg
	Protein	8 g	Calcium	199 mg

Cough and Sore Throat Soother

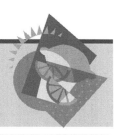

We often drink this addictive beauty just because it's so good. The ingredients are well known to ease sore throats and coughs. Honey lubricates the throat, and ginger is anti-microbial. The vitamin C and minerals help strengthen your immune system to fight the cold that can irritate the throat.

1/2 freshly brewed green tea, cooled
1 tsp. fresh orange zest
1/2 cup navel orange, peeled and diced
1/2 tsp. fresh lemon zest
1/2 lemon, peeled and seeded
3/4 tsp. fresh ginger root, chopped
1 T. dried egg white powder
2 tsp. honey

Zest the fruit before peeling. Place all ingredients into blender and mix until smooth. This is a shake rather than a smoothie. Substitute crushed ice for the tea for a slushier consistency.

Lemon is touted as a leader in neutralizing a kidney patient's acidic state, perhaps rivaling baking soda. Citrus flavonoids have powerful biological properties shown to play an important role in treating high cholesterol, insulin resistance, obesity, and atherosclerosis.[11] Regularly enjoy lemons and oranges.

Nutrient Values				
	Calories	116	Potassium	253 mg
	Fat	0 g	Phosphorus	29 mg
	Fiber	2 g	Sodium	91 mg
	Protein	7 g	Calcium	50 mg

Blood Pressure Easer

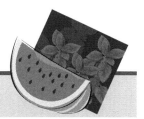

Ruby-red watermelon is an excellent source of vitamin C and antioxidants, including lycopene, and aids in blood pressure control. Yogurt, oats, and mint have anti-inflammatory properties, important for kidney patients.

1 cup watermelon, cubed
2 fresh mint leaves
1/4 cup oat flakes (we use old-fashioned oats)
1/2 single-serving container nonfat, plain Greek yogurt (3 ounces)
1/2 cup crushed ice

Place all ingredients into blender and mix until smooth.

Up to 94% of dialysis patients have high blood pressure. In several small studies, watermelon reduced arterial stiffness and blood pressure in people with either prehypertension or hypertension.[12] That's a good reason to love this melon.

Nutrient Values	Calories	173	Potassium	364 mg
	Fat	2 g	Phosphorus	215 mg
	Fiber	3 g	Sodium	34 mg
	Protein	12 g	Calcium	116 mg

Peaches & Cream

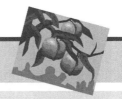

This smoothie snack quenches that peach pie urge. Peaches pack 10 different vitamins and several minerals for few calories. Phenolic compounds in peaches show anti-obesity and anti-inflammatory effects, good in CKD. Yogurt contains live cultures that promote intestinal health.

1/2 cup water or freshly brewed green tea, cooled
3/4 cup frozen peach slices, unsweetened
1/2 single-serving container nonfat, plain Greek yogurt (3 ounces)
1/4 tsp. ground nutmeg
1/2 tsp. pure vanilla extract

Place all ingredients into blender and mix until smooth.

Kidney patients at any CKD stage suffer depression at 4 times the rate of the general population. Nearly 50% of dialysis patients are depressed. Studies link depression in dialysis with increased hospitalizations, shortened survival, and reduced quality of life.[13] Ask for help. Treatment lessens depression nearly 80% of the time.

Nutrient Values				
	Calories	104	Potassium	344 mg
	Fat	1 g	Phosphorus	139 mg
	Fiber	2 g	Sodium	31 mg
	Protein	10 g	Calcium	102 mg

Vitamin C Daily Dose

The pineapple provides 100% of the recommended daily allowance of vitamin C, a vitamin important in avoiding anemia and increasing survival in dialysis. Cardamom is an Ayurvedic healing spice shown to ease stomach and bowel distress, as does yogurt. Flax is heart-healthy. You'll be pleasantly surprised by the fragrant taste of this smoothie.

1 cup frozen pineapple chunks, unsweetened
1 single-serve container nonfat, plain Greek yogurt (170 g)
1 T. ground flax seeds
1/4 tsp. cardamom
1/2 cup water or freshly brewed green tea, cooled

Place all ingredients into blender and mix until smooth. Add additional liquid if you prefer a thinner consistency.

Vitamin C deficiency is unnecessarily common in dialysis patients. It is often lost during dialysis treatments, and dietary limitations inadvertently result in exclusion of produce high in vitamin C. Yet, dialysis places an extra demand on the need for vitamin C. Research shows that vitamin C in dialysis aids absorption of iron to reduce anemia, lessen chronic inflammation, extend survival, and lower periodontal (gum) disease risk.[14]

Nutrient Values				
	Calories	171	Potassium	363 mg
	Fat	4 g	Phosphorus	174 mg
	Fiber	4 g	Sodium	35 mg
	Protein	11 g	Calcium	135 mg

Easing Hypertension

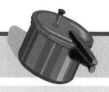

Beets have the impressive ability to lower blood pressure within hours of consuming them. Blueberries and low fat dairy are copycats, also easing pressure. Enjoy this smoothie as your blood vessels relax.

1/4 cup 100% beet juice, unsweetened (or use raw or cooked beets)
1/2 cup water
1 cup frozen blueberries, unsweetened
1/3 cup 1% lowfat cottage cheese
1 tsp. fresh lemon juice
4 fresh basil leaves, torn

Place all ingredients into blender and mix until smooth.

Hypertension is widespread in CKD. Regular consumption of nitrates found in green vegetables and beets may help ease blood pressure. In a recent review of 16 trials involving 254 participants, daily beetroot juice and nitrate supplementation were associated with a significant decrease in systolic blood pressure.[15]

Nutrient Values	Calories	150	Potassium	282 mg
	Fat	1 g	Phosphorus	135 mg
	Fiber	7 g	Sodium	337 mg
	Protein	10 g	Calcium	79 mg

Antioxidant Heart Power

Blueberries, strawberries, mint, and green tea are rich in antioxidants, making this smoothie cardiovascular and blood pressure protective, anti-inflammatory, and memory enhancing. Blueberries rank among the top disease-fighting foods, thanks to their anthocyanins. We love organic, wild blueberries.

1/2 cup frozen blueberries, unsweetened
1/2 cup frozen strawberries, unsweetened
1 single-serve container nonfat, plain Greek yogurt (170 g.)
2 mint leaves
1/2 cup water or freshly brewed green tea, cooled

Place all ingredients into blender and mix until smooth.

A diet rich in antioxidants may reduce the high cardiovascular risk in dialysis. In a 10-year study of 32,561 women, those consuming the highest levels of antioxidants (7 servings of fruits/vegetables per day) had a 20% lowered risk of heart attack compared to those getting only 2.4 servings a day.[16] Enjoy 2 fruit servings in this smoothie, and add another smoothie during the day.

Nutrient Values	Calories	166	Potassium	399 mg
	Fat	1 g	Phosphorus	249 mg
	Fiber	5 g	Sodium	65 mg
	Protein	18 g	Calcium	211 mg

Orange Sherbet with a Healing Plus

Pineapple contains bromelain, an anti-inflammatory enzyme that may help to reduce pain and internal inflammation. Pineapple is also a good source of vitamin C to strengthen the immune system. In this smoothie, it is a delicious treat.

1/2 cup water
1/2 cup frozen pineapple chunks, unsweetened
1 scoop vanilla whey protein powder (we use Biochem)
1/2 tsp. fresh lime juice
1 tsp. zest from orange
1/2 cup orange sherbet

Place all ingredients, except the sherbet, into blender and mix until smooth. Add the sherbet, blending to make a shake. Umm, good!

Metabolic syndrome (MS) is common in CKD. Researchers followed 163 non-diabetic peritoneal dialysis patients. The 52% with MS were significantly heavier; had higher blood pressure, triglyceride, and total cholesterol levels; and had lower LDL levels than PD patients without MS. Survival of patients with MS was also significantly lower.[17] Consuming more fruits and vegetables (think, smoothies) and limiting saturated fats and sugars can help relieve MS.

Nutrient Values				
	Calories	206	Potassium	212 mg
	Fat	2 g	Phosphorus	63 mg
	Fiber	2 g	Sodium	57 mg
	Protein	11 g	Calcium	103 mg

Veggie Salad Punch

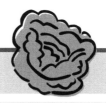

Weird ingredients, but this drink tastes delicious, and vegetables rank tops as health-promoting foods. Their antioxidants and phytochemicals help kidney patients reduce metabolic acidosis, maintain proper weight, eliminate damaging internal inflammation, lower blood pressure, decrease cardiovascular risk, and so on. Vegetables are heart-friendly sources of protein.

1/4 cup fresh cucumber with peel, diced
1/2 cup frozen pineapple chunks
1 tsp. fresh lemon juice
1 cup red leaf lettuce, chopped
1/4 cup fresh cabbage, chopped
1/5 package Nasoya extra firm tofu (about 1/2 cup)
1/2 cup water or freshly brewed green tea, cooled
2 fresh basil leaves
1 tsp. extra virgin olive oil

Place all ingredients except lettuce and cabbage in blender, and mix until smooth. Add the lettuce and cabbage, blending until smooth. Add additional liquid if needed.

Pilot studies are ongoing to change the traditional dialysis diet to one more plant-centered. Current dialysis diets stress animal protein (full of saturated fat). A re-evaluation of plant-based protein shows it is just as adequate as meat as a protein source and is substantially more heart-healthy. Phytates in plant protein are shown to decrease availability of phosphorus (that's good in CKD).[18] Talk with your dietitian about fitting more produce into your diet.

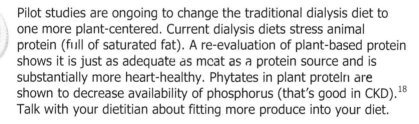

Nutrient Values	Calories	171	Potassium	233 mg
	Fat	9 g	Phosphorus	136 mg
	Fiber	3 g	Sodium	20 mg
	Protein	9 g	Calcium	247 mg

Echoes of Apple Pie

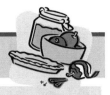

Phytochemicals in apples and cherries seem to help repair and protect against cellular damage that plays a negative role in a number of chronic diseases, including CKD. The fruits are a good source of soluble fiber, which helps to reduce cholesterol levels, improve heart health, and maintain a healthy digestive tract.

1/2 cup apple with peel, chopped and core removed
1/2 cup frozen sour cherries, unsweetened
1/2 cup 100% apple juice, unsweetened
1/2 tsp. ground cinnamon
1/4 cup oat flakes
1 scoop vanilla whey powder (we use Biochem)

Place all ingredients in blender and mix until smooth.

An apple a day really is good for the heart, recent research reports. Study participants who ate one apple a day for four weeks had reduced blood levels of oxidized low-density lipoprotein (LDL), or bad cholesterol, compared to non-apple eaters.[19] LDL reduction can significantly decrease risk for atherosclerosis (hardening of the arteries), a decrease important in kidney disease.

Nutrient Values	Calories	260	Potassium	411 mg
	Fat	2 g	Phosphorus	137 mg
	Fiber	6 g	Sodium	30 mg
	Protein	14 g	Calcium	96 mg

Strawberry Shake

This smoothie is a fun way to sneak in some beta-carotene from carrots, which converts to vitamin A in your body. Strawberries, with their polyphenols, rank among the top 20 fruits in antioxidant capacity and are packed with vitamin C and fiber.

1/2 cup water
1/2 cup frozen strawberries, unsweetened
1/4 cup steamed, raw, or frozen carrot slices
1 scoop vanilla whey powder
1 tsp. pure vanilla extract
1/4 tsp. ground cinnamon
1/2 cup strawberry sherbet

Place all ingredients except sherbet in blender and mix until smooth. Blend in sherbet.

Want to improve your quality of life? Hop on line and join facebook groups. Social networking is shown to reduce depression in dialysis and improve cognitive function, education, sleep, and quality of life.[20] During dialysis sessions is a great time to use that tablet.

Nutrient Values				
	Calories	215	Potassium	312 mg
	Fat	2 g	Phosphorus	77 mg
	Fiber	4 g	Sodium	80 mg
	Protein	12 g	Calcium	125 mg

Cherry-Berry Cheesecake

Cherries help reduce uric acid levels to ease the pain of gout and arthritis and reduce acidosis. Their polyphenols are known to keep blood vessels open and flexible. Cherries, strawberries, and cinnamon contain phytochemicals to help relieve metabolic inflammation and lower blood pressure. On top of all this, the fruits taste great!

1/2 cup frozen red sour cherries, unsweetened
1/2 cup fresh strawberries, halved
1 full graham cracker sheet, broken into blender
1/2 tsp. pure vanilla extract
1/2 tsp. ground cinnamon
1/4 cup ricotta cheese, part skim milk
1/2 cup water

Place all ingredients in blender and mix until smooth and creamy.

 Exercise helps prevent and treat the protein and energy wasting so widespread in dialysis.[21] The amount of exercise (walking) can be as little as 15 minutes a day, 3 times a week to see an uplift in mood, improved muscle response, increased energy, better nutritional status, and more effective dialysis sessions.

Nutrient Values				
	Calories	216	Potassium	312 mg
	Fat	7 g	Phosphorus	151 mg
	Fiber	4 g	Sodium	131 mg
	Protein	9 g	Calcium	207 mg

APPENDIX 1

Prognosis of CKD by GFR and albuminuria category

Prognosis of CKD by GFR and Albuminuria Categories: KDIGO 2012			Persistent albuminuria categories Description and range		
			A1 Normal to mildly increased <30 mg/g <3 mg/mmol	A2 Moderately increased 30-300 mg/g 3-30 mg/mmol	A3 Severely increased >300 mg/g >30 mg/mmol
GFR categories (ml/min/ 1.73 m²) Description and range	G1	Normal or high	≥90			
	G2	Mildly decreased	60-89			
	G3a	Mildly to moderately decreased	45-59			
	G3b	Moderately to severely decreased	30-44			
	G4	Severely decreased	15-29			
	G5	Kidney failure	<15			

Green: low risk (if no other markers of kidney disease, no CKD); Yellow: moderately increased risk; Orange: high risk; Red, very high risk.

APPENDIX 2

DASH Eating Plan – 2000 Calories Per Day

Food Group	Amount/Frequency	Examples of Portions
Fruits	2-2½ Cups Daily	½ Cup: 1 med. fresh fruit, 16 grapes, ½ cup fresh, canned or frozen, ¼ cup dried, 4 oz. 100% juice
Vegetables	2-2½ Cups Daily	½ Cup: 1 cup leafy greens, ½ cup raw, canned* or frozen, or 4 oz. 100% juice
Fat-free or Lowfat Dairy	2-3 Cups Daily	1 Cup: 8 oz. milk, 8 oz. yogurt, 1½ oz. lowfat, fat-free or reduced fat natural cheese, 2 oz. lowfat or fat-free processed cheese
Whole Grains	6-8 Ounces Daily	1 Ounce: 1 oz. sliced bread, ½ cup cooked rice or pasta, ½-1¼ cups dry cereal*
Lean Meat, Fish, Poultry	6 or less Ounces Daily	1 Ounce: 1 oz. cooked beef, fish or chicken, or 1 egg. (Note: 3 ounces roughly equals a deck of cards)
Nuts, Seeds and Legumes	4-5 Times Weekly	1/3 cup or 1½ oz. nuts, 2 T. peanut butter, ½ oz. seeds, ½ cup cooked dry beans, peas or lentils
Oils	2-3 Teaspoons Daily (Use sparingly)	1 Teaspoon: 1 tsp. soft margarine, 1 T. low-fat mayo, 2 T. low-fat salad dressing, 1 tsp. vegetable oil
Added Sugar	5 Tablespoons per Week	1 Tablespoon: 1 T. sugar, 1 T. jelly or jam, ½ cup sorbet and ices, 1 cup lemonade
Sodium	2300 Milligrams per Day	2300 mg sodium = 1 teaspoon salt. For kidney patients, the limit is 1500 mg. sodium
Alcohol	Use Sparingly	1 drink = 12 oz. beer, 5 oz. wine, 1.5 oz. spirits (Men: 2 or less per day; Women: 1 or less per day)

*Check nutrient facts label

Endnotes

Chapter 1 - Respect Those Beans

Chronic Kidney Disease 101

[1] U.S. Renal Data System, USRDS 2013 Annual Data Report: Atlas of Chronic Kidney Disease and End-Stage Renal Disease in the United States, National Institutes of Health, National Institute of Diabetes and Digestive and Kidney Disease, Bethesda, MD. 2013;Vol.1, Ch.1.

[2] Grams ME, Chow EK, Segev DL, Coresh J. "Lifetime incidence of CKD stages 3-5 in the United States." *Am J Kidney Dis.* 2013;62(2):245-252.

[3] Grubbs V, Plantinga LC, Tuot DS, et al. "Americans' use of dietary supplements that are potentially harmful in CKD." *Am J Kidney Dis.* 2013 May;61(5):739-47.

[4] U.S. Renal Data System, USRDS 2013 Annual Data Report: Atlas of Chronic Kidney Disease and End-Stage Renal Disease in the United States, National Institutes of Health, National Institute of Diabetes and Digestive and Kidney Disease, Bethesda, MD. 2013;Vol.1, Ch.1.

[5] National Kidney Foundation. Kidney Disease: Improving Global Outcomes (KDIGO) CKD Work Group. KDIGO 2012 Clinical Practice Guidelines for the Evaluation and Management of Chronic Kidney Disease. *Kidney Int., Suppl.* 2013;3:1-150.

[6] Id.

[7] Turin TC, Tonelli M, Mannis BJ, et al. "Proteinuria and life expectancy." *Am J Kidney Dis.* 2013 Apr;61(4):646-8.

[8] National Kidney Foundation. Kidney Disease: Improving Global Outcomes (KDIGO) CKD Work Group. KDIGO 2012 Clinical Practice Guidelines for the Evaluation and Management of Chronic Kidney Disease. *Kidney Int., Suppl.* 2013;3:1-150.

[9] Hajhosseiny R, Khavandi K, Goldsmith DJ. "Cardiovascular disease in chronic kidney disease." *Int J Clin Pract.* 2013;67(1):14-31.

[10] Choudhury D, Levi M. "Kidney aging--inevitable or preventable?" *Nat Rev Nephrol.* 2011 Aug 9;7(12):706-17.

[11] U.S. Renal Data System, USRDS 2013 Annual Data Report: Atlas of Chronic Kidney Disease and End-Stage Renal Disease in the United States, National Institutes of Health, National Institute of Diabetes and Digestive and Kidney Disease, Bethesda, MD. 2013;Vol.1, Ch.1.

[12] Choudhury D, Levi M. "Kidney aging--inevitable or preventable?" *Nat Rev Nephrol.* 2011 Aug 9;7(12):706-17.

Kidneys and Heart: Partners in Distress

[1] Muntner P, Judd SE, Gao, L, et al. "Cardiovascular risk factors in CKD associated with both ESRD and mortality." *J Am Soc Nephrol,* 2013 Jun;24(7):1159-65.

[2] National Kidney Foundation. "Kidney Disease: Improving Global Outcomes (KDIGO) CKD Work Group. KDIGO 2012 Clinical Practice Guidelines for the Evaluation and Management of Chronic Kidney Disease." *Kidney Int. Suppl.* 2013;3:1-150.

[3] Moody WE, Edwards NC, Chue CD, et al. "Arterial disease in chronic kidney disease." *Heart.* 2013;99(6):365-372.

[4] Salmon AH, Ferguson JK, Burford JL, et al. "Loss of the endothelial glycocalyx links albuminuria and vascular dysfunction." *J Am Soc Nephrol.* 2012 Aug:23(8):1339-50.

[5] Hajhosseiny R, Khavandi K, Goldsmith DJ. "Cardiovascular disease in chronic kidney disease." *Int J Clin Pract.* 2013;67(1):14-31.

[6] U.S. Renal Data System, USRDS 2013 Annual Data Report: Atlas of Chronic Kidney Disease and End-Stage Renal Disease in the United States, National Institutes of Health, National Institute of Diabetes and Digestive and Kidney Disease, Bethesda, MD. 2013;Vol.2, Ch.4:247.

[7]Muntner P, Judd SE, Gao, L, et al. "Cardiovascular risk factors in CKD associate with both ESRD and mortality." *J Am Soc Nephrol.* 2013 Jun;24(7):1159-65.

[8]Ricardo AC, Madero M, Yang W, et al. "Adherence to a healthy lifestyle and all-cause mortality in CKD." *Clin. J Am Soc Nephrol.* 2013 Apr;8(4):602-9.

[9]Sacco RL. "The new American Heart Association 2020 goal: achieving ideal cardiovascular health." *J Cardiovasc.* 2011 Apr;12(4):255-7.

[10]Dehghan M, Mente A, Teo KK, et al. "Relationship between healthy diet and risk of cardiovascular disease among patients on drug therapies for secondary prevention: a prospective cohort study of 31,546 high-risk individuals from 40 countries." *Circulation.* 2012 Dec 4;126(23):2705-12.

Chapter 2 - Kidney Disease: Largely Food-Based

Diabetes: Unnecessarily Rampant

[1]American Diabetes Association. Diabetes Basics: http://www.diabetes.org/diabetes-basics/statistics/?loc=db-slabnav.

[2]Couser WG, Remuzzi G, Mendis S, Tonelli M. "The contribution of chronic kidney disease to global burden of major noncommunicable diseases." *Kidney Int.* 2011;80(12):1258-1270.

[3]Afkarian M, Sachs MC, Kestenbaum B, et al. "Kidney disease and increased mortality risk in type 2 diabetes." *J Am Soc Nephrol.* 2013 Feb;24(2):302-8.

[4]Plantinga LC, Crews DC, Coresh J, et al. "Prevalence of chronic kidney disease in US adults with undiagnosed diabetes or prediabetes." *Clin J Am Soc Nephrol.* 2010 Apr;5(4):673-82.

[5]Centers for Disease Control and Prevention. Fast Facts: http://www.cdc.gov/nchs/fastats/deaths.htm.

[6]American Diabetes Association. Food and Fitness: http://www.diabetes.org/food-and-fitness/food/what-can-i-eat/what-can-i-drink.html.

[7]Summary of revisions for the 2013 clinical practice recommendations. *Diabetes Care.* 2013 Jan;36 Suppl 1:S3. doi: 10.2337/dc13-S003; National Kidney Foundation. KDOQITM Clinical Practice Guidelines and Clinical Practice Recommendations for Diabetes and Chronic Kidney Disease. *Am J Kidney Dis.* 49:S1-S180,2007 (supp 2), Guideline 5.

[8]InterAct Consortium. "Consumption of sweet beverages and type 2 diabetes incidence in European adults: results from EPIC-InterAct." *Diabetologia.* 2013 Jul;56(7):1520-30.

[9]Summary of revisions for the 2013 clinical practice recommendations. *Diabetes Care.* 2013 Jan;36 Suppl 1:S3. doi: 10.2337/dc13-S003; National Kidney Foundation. KDOQITM Clinical Practice Guidelines and Clinical Practice Recommendations for Diabetes and Chronic Kidney Disease. *Am J Kidney Dis.* 49:S1-S180,2007 (supp 2), Guideline 5.

[10]Christensen AS, Viggers L, Hasselstrom K, Gregersen S. "Effect of fruit restriction on glycemic control in patients with type 2 diabetes--a randomized trial." *Nutr J.* 2013 Mar 5;12:29.

Blood Pressure: Help it Head South

[1]U.S. Renal Data System, USRDS 2013 Annual Data Report: Atlas of Chronic Kidney Disease and End-Stage Renal Disease in the United States, National Institutes of Health, National Institute of Diabetes and Digestive and Kidney Disease, Bethesda, MD. 2013;Vol.1, Ch.1:48.

[2]Id. at Vol.1, Ch.1:54.

[3]Centers of Disease Control and Prevention, http://www.cdc.gov/bloodpressure/; Go AS, Mozaffarean D, Roger VL, et al. "Heart disease and stroke statistics--2013 update: a report from the American Heart Association." *Circulation.* 2013;127:143-152.

[4]Egan BM, Li J, Qanungo S, Wolfman TE. "Blood pressure and cholesterol control in hypertensive hypercholesterolemic patients: National health and nutrition examination surveys 1988 to 2010." *Circulation.* 2013 Jul 2;128(1):29-41.

[5]U.S. Renal Data System, USRDS 2013 Annual Data Report: Atlas of Chronic Kidney Disease and End-Stage Renal Disease in the United States, National Institutes of Health, National Institute of Diabetes and Digestive and Kidney Disease, Bethesda, MD. 2013;Vol.1, Ch.4.

[6]National Kidney Foundation. Kidney Disease: Improving Global Outcomes (KDIGO), CKD Work Group. KDIGO 2012 Clinical Practice Guidelines for the Evaluation and Management of Chronic Kidney Disease. *Kidney Inter. Suppl.* 2013;3:73.

[7]Kovesdy CP, Bleyer AJ, Molnaret MZ, et al. "Blood pressure and mortality in U.S. veterans with chronic kidney disease: a cohort study."*Ann Intern Med.* 2013;159:233-242.

[8]U.S. Renal Data System, USRDS 2013 Annual Data Report: Atlas of Chronic Kidney Disease and End-Stage Renal Disease in the United States, National Institutes of Health, National Institute of Diabetes and Digestive and Kidney Disease, Bethesda, MD. 2013;Vol.1, Ch.4.

[9]American Heart Association. Prevention and Treatment of High Blood Pressure: http://www.heart.org/HEARTORG/Conditions/HighBloodPressure/PreventionTreatmentofHighBloodPressure/Prevention-Treatment-of-High-Blood Pressure_UCM_002054_Article.jsp.

[10]Gilchrist M, Winyard PG, Alzawa K, et al. "Effect of dietary nitrate on blood pressure, endothelial function, and insulin sensitivity in type 2 diabetes." *Free Radic Biol Med.* 2013 Jul;60:89-97.

That Spare Tire: A Separate Creature

[1]Centers for Disease Control and Prevention. Obesity Facts. http://www.cdc.gov/obesity/data/facts.html.

[2]Couser WG, Remuzzi G, Mendis S, Tonelli M. "The contribution of chronic kidney disease to the global burden of major noncommunicable diseases." *Kidney Int.* 2011;80(12):1258-1270.

[3]Masters RK, Reither EN, Powers DA, et al. "The impact of obesity on US mortality levels: the importance of age and cohort factors in population estimates." *Am J Public Health.* 2013 Oct;103(10):1895-1901.

[4]Kwakernaak AJ, Zelle DM, Bakker SJ, Navis G. "Central body fat distribution associates with unfavorable renal hemodynamics independent of body mass index." *J Am Soc Nephrol.* 2013 May;24(6):987-94.

[5]Stenvinkel P, Ikizier TA, Mallamaci F, Zoccali C. "Obesity and nephrology: results of a knowledge and practice pattern survey." *Nephrol Dial Transplant.* 2013 Nov;28 Suppl 4:iv99-104.

[6]Cordeiro AC, Qureshi AR, Lindholm B, et al. "Visceral fat and coronary artery calcification in patients with chronic kidney disease." *Nephrol Dial Transplant.* 2013 Jul 5.

[7]Ridaura VK, Faith JJ, Rey FE, et al. "Gut microbes from twins discordant for obesity modulate metabolism in mice." *Science.* 2013 Sep 6;341(6150):1241214.

[8]Source: National Heart, Lung, and Blood Institute

[9]Singh AK, Kari JA. "Metabolic syndrome and chronic kidney disease." *Curr Opin Nephrol Hypertens.* 2013 Mar;22(2):198-203.

[10]Agarwal S, Shlipak MG, Kramer H, et al. "The association of chronic kidney disease and metabolic syndrome with incident cardiovascular events: multiethnic study of atherosclerosis." *Cardio Res Pract.* 2012;2012:806102.

[11]Akbaraly TN, Singh-Manoux A, Tabak AG, et al. "Overall diet history and reversibility of the metabolic syndrome over 15 years: the Whitehall II prospective cohort study." *Diabetes Care.* 2010 Nov;33(11):2339-41.

Sugar: Not So Sweet for Health

[1] Lustig RH. (2013) *Fat chance: beating the odds against sugar, processed food, obesity, and diabetes.* New York:Hudson Street Press.

[2] Goran MI, Ulljaszek SJ, Ventura EE. "High fructose corn syrup and diabetes prevalence: a global perspective." *Glob Public Health.* 2013;8(1):55-64.
http://www.ers.usda.gov/publications/sssm-sugar-and-sweeteners-outlook/sssm286.aspx#.UeMY9eDR1SU

[3] Aeberli I, Houchuli M, Gerber PA, et al. "Moderate amounts of fructose consumption impair insulin sensitivity in healthy young men: a randomized controlled trial." *Diabetes Care.* 2013 Jan;36(1):150-6.

[4] Lim SS, Vos T, Flaxman AD. "A comparative risk assessment of burden of diseases and injury attributable to 67 risk factors and risk factor clusters in 21 regions, 1990-2010: a systematic analysis for the Global Burden of Disease Study 2010. " *Lancet.* 2012 Dec 15;380:9859;2224-60.

[5] Saldana TM, Basso O, Darden R, Sandler DP. "Carbonated beverages and chronic kidney disease." *Epidemiology.* 2007 Jul;18(4):501-6.

[6] Ferraro PM, Taylor EN, Gambaro G, Curhan GC. "Soda and other beverages and the risk of kidney stones." *Clin J Am Soc Nephrol.* 2013 Aug;8(8):1389-95.

[7] Karalius VP, Shoham DA. "Dietary sugar and artificial sweetener intake and chronic kidney disease: a review." *Adv Chronic kidney Dis.* 2013 Mar;20(2):157-64.

[8] Brymora A, Flisinski M, Johnson RJ, et al. "Low-fructose diet lowers blood pressure and inflammation in patients with chronic kidney disease." *Nephrol Dial Transplant.* 2012 Feb;27(2):608-12.

[9] Lawrence de Koning, Malik VS, Kellogg MD, Eric B. Rimm, et al. "Sweetened beverage consumption, incident coronary heart disease and biomarkers of risk in men." *Circulation. 2012* Apr 10;125(14):1735-41.

[10] Richelsen B. "Sugar-sweetened beverages and cardio-metabolic disease risks." *Curr Opin Nutr Metab Care.* 2013 Jul;16(4):478-84.

[11] Center for Disease Control and Prevention. cdc.gov/nchs/data/databriefs/db71.htm

[12] Ibid.

[13] Krebs-Smith SM, Guenther PM, Subar AF, et al. "Americans do not meet dietary recommendations." *J.Nutr.* 2010 Oct;140(10):1832-8.

[14] Johnson RK, Appel LJ, Brands M, et al. "Dietary sugars intake and cardiovascular health: a scientific statement from the American Heart Association." *Circulation.* 2009 Sep 15;120(11):1011-20.

[15] Swithers SE. "Artificial sweeteners produce the counterintuitive effect of inducing metabolic derangements." *Trends Endocrinol Metab.* 2013 Sept;24(9):431-41.

Fats - The Good, The Bad, The Ugly

[1] Stanhope KL, Bremer AA, Medici V, et al. "Consumption of fructose and high fructose corn syrup increase postprandial triglycerides, LDL-cholesterol, and apolipoprotein-B in young men and women." *J Clin Endocrinol Metab.* 2011 Oct;96(10):E1596-605.

[2] Id.

[3] Turner JM, Bauer C, Abramowitz MK, el al. "Treatment of chronic kidney disease." *Kidney Int.* 2012;81(4):351-362.

[4] Ni J, Wang CX, Liu J, et al. "Activation of renin-angiotensin system is involved in dyslipidemia-mediated renal injuries in apolipoprotein E knockout mice and HK-2 cells." *Lipids Health Dis.* 2013 Apr 9;12(1):49.

[5]Sandu S, Wiebe N, Fried LF, et al. "Statins for improving renal outcomes: a meta-analysis." *J Am Soc. Nephrol.* 2006; 17:2006-2016.

[6]Chung YH, Lee YC, Chang CH, et al. "Statins of high versus low cholesterol-lowering efficacy and the development of severe renal failure." *Pharmacoepidemiol Drug Saf.* 2013 June;22(6):583-92; Baryiski M, Nikfar S, Mikhailidis DP, et al. "Statins decrease all-cause mortality only in CKD patients not requiring dialysis therapy - a meta-analysis of 11 randomized controlled trials involving 21,295 participants." *Pharmacol Res.* 2013 Jun;72:35-44.

Setting Our Kids Up for CKD

[1]U.S. Renal Data System, USRDS 2013 Annual Data Report: Atlas of Chronic Kidney Disease and End-Stage Renal Disease in the United States, National Institutes of Health, National Institute of Diabetes and Digestive and Kidney Disease, Bethesda, MD. 2013;Vol.2, Ch.8.

[2]Centers for Disease Control and Prevention. Overweight and Obesity. http://www.cdc.gov/obesity/data/childhood.html.

[3]Hamman RF, Pettitt DJ, Dabelea D, et al. "Estimates of the burden of diabetes in United States Youth in 2009." American Diabetes Association 2012 Scientific Sessions; June 9, 2012; Philadelphia, PA. Abstract 1369-P.

[4]TODAT Study Group. "Rapid rise in hypertension and nephropathy in youth with type 2 diabetes: the TODAY clinical trial." *Diabetes Care.* 2013 Jun;36(6):1735-41.

[5]Tran CL, Ehrmann BJ, Messer KL, et al. "Recent trends in healthcare utilization among children and adolescents with hypertension in the United States." *Hypertension.* 2012;60:296-302.

[6]Id.

[7]Hamman RF, Pettitt DJ, Dabelea D, et al. "Estimates of the burden of diabetes in United States Youth in 2009." American Diabetes Association 2012 Scientific Sessions; June 9, 2012; Philadelphia, PA. Abstract 1369-P.

[8]Grams ME, Chow EK, Segev DL, Coresh J. "Lifetime incidence of CKD stages 3-5 in the United States." *Am J Kidney Dis.* 2013;62(2):245-252.

[9]Vivante A, Golan E, Tzur D, et al. "Body mass index in 1.2 million adolescents and risk for end-stage renal disease." *Arch Intern Med.* 2012 Nov 26;172(21):1644-50.

[10]Yang Q, Zhang Z, Kuklina EV. "Sodium intake and blood pressure among US children and adolescents." *Pediatrics.* 2012 Oct;130(4):611-9.

[11]Ervin RB, Kit BK, Carroll MD, Ogden CL. "Consumption of added sugar among U.S. children and adolescents, 2005–2008." NCHS data brief, no 87. Hyattsville, MD: National Center for Health Statistics. 2012.

[12]Deboer MD, Scharf RJ, Demmer RT. "Sugar-sweetened beverages and weight gain in 2- to 5-year-old children." *Pediatrics.* 2012 Oct;130(4):611-9.

[13]American Academy of Pediatrics. Council on Communications and Media. Policy Statement--Children, Adolescents, Obesity, and the Media. http://pediatrics.aappublications.org/content/early/2011/06/23/peds.2011-1066.full.pdf+html.

[14]Moore LL, Bradlee ML, Singer MR, et al. "Dietary Approaches to Stop Hypertension (DASH) eating pattern and risk of elevated blood pressure in adolescent girls." *Br J Nutr.* 2012 Nov 14;108(9):1678-85.

Chapter 3 - Eats Kidneys Love

DASH for Health

[1]National Kidney Foundation. KDOQI Clinical Practice Guidelines and Clinical Practice Recommendations for Diabetes and Chronic Kidney Disease. *Am J Kidney Dis.* 49:S1-S180, 2007 (suppl 2), Guideline 5.

[2]Id.

[3]Appel LJ, Moore TJ, Obarzanek E, et al. "A clinical trial of the effects of dietary patterns on blood pressure. DASH Collaborative Research Group." *N Engl J Med.* 1997;336(16):1117-24.

[4]For a listing of numerous studies on health benefits of the DASH diet, see http://www.dashdiet.org/dash_diet_research.asp.

[5]Chang A, Van Horn L, Jacobs DR Jr, et al. "Lifestyle-related factors, obesity, and incident microalbuminuria: The CARDIA (Coronary Artery Risk Development in Young Adults) Study." *Am J Kidney Dis.* 2013 Apr 10. pii:S0272-6386(13)00574-X; Lin J, Fung TT, Hu FB, Curhan GC. "Association of dietary patterns with albuminuria and kidney function decline in older white women: a subgroup analysis from the Nurses' Health Study." *Am J Kidney Dis.* 2011 Feb;57(2):245-54.

[6]National Kidney Foundation 2011 Clinical Meetings: Abstract 61. presented April 28, 2011.

[7]Khatri M, et al. "The impact of a Mediterranean style diet on kidney function." *Am Soc Nephrol.* 2013. Abstract OR052.

Renal Diet: A Confusing Label

[1]National Kidney Foundation. Kidney Disease: Improving Global Outcomes (KDIGO) CKD Work Group. KDIGO 2012 Clinical Practice Guidelines for the Evaluation and Management of Chronic Kidney Disease. *Kidney Int., Suppl.* 2013;3:1-150.

Antioxidants: Health Superheroes

[1]Eg., Birch-Machin MA, Russell EV, Latimer JA. "Mitochondrial DNA damage as a biomarker for ultraviolet radiation exposure and oxidative stress." *Br. J. Dermatol.* 2013 Jul; 169 Suppl 2:9-14.

[2]Eg., Fishman AI, Green D, Lynch A, et al. "Preventive effects of specific antioxidant on oxidative renal cell injury associated with renal cell formation." *Urology.* 2013 Aug;82(2):489.

[3]Eg., Aminzadeh MA, Nicholas SB, Norris KC, Vaziri ND. "Role of Impaired Nrf2 activation in the pathogenesis of oxidative stress and inflammation in C tubulo-interstitial nephropathy." *Nephrol Dial Transplant.* 2013 Aug;28(8):2038-45.

[4]The American Heart Association, National Kidney Foundation, and other leading authorities do not advocate supplements unless specifically prescribed by a doctor.

Phytochemicals: Key to Better Health

[1]Huang X, Jimenez-Moleon JJ, Lindholm B, et al. "Mediterranean diet, kidney function, and mortality in men with CKD." *Clin J Am Soc Nephrol.* 2013 Sep;8(9):1548-55; Goraya N, Simoni J, Jo C-H, Wesson DE. "A comparison of treating metabolic acidosis in CKD stage 4 hypertensive kidney disease with fruits and vegetables or sodium bicarbonate." *Clin J Am Soc Nephrol.* 2013 Mar;8(3):371-81.

[2]Huang T, Yang B, Zheng J, et al. "Cardiovascular disease mortality and cancer incidence in vegetarians: a meta-analysis and systematic review." *Ann Nutr Metab.* 2012;60(4):233-40; Lo YT, Chang VH, Wahiqvist ML, et al. "Spending on vegetable and fruit consumption could reduce all-cause mortality among older adults." *Nutr J.* 2012 Dec 19;11:113.

Fiber: Kidney Disease Fighter

[1]Díaz-López A, Bulló M, Basora J, Martínez-González MÁ, et al. "Cross-sectional associations between macronutrient intake and chronic kidney disease in a population at high cardiovascular risk." *Clin Nutr.* 2013 Aug;32(4):606-12.

[2]Evenepoel P, Meijers BK. "Dietary fiber and protein:nutritional therapy in chronic kidney disease and beyond." *Kidney Int.* 2012 Feb;81(3):227-9

[3] Gopinath B, Harris DC, Flood VM, Burlutsky G, et al. "Dietary fiber and protein: nutritional therapy in chronic kidney disease and beyond." *J Nutr.* 2011 Mar;141(3):433-9.

[4] Threapleton DE, Greenwood DC, Evans CE, et al. "Dietary fiber intake and risk of stroke: a systematic review and meta-analysis." *Stroke.* 2013 May;44(5):1360-8.

[5] U.S. Department of Health and Human Services, U.S. Department of Agriculture. Dietary Guidelines for Americans 2010. Washington, DC: Government Publishing Office, 2010. Ch.4:40-41.

Chapter 4 - Slowing Kidney Damage With Produce

Acidosis: Internal Burn

[1] Goraya N, Wesson DE. "Dietary management of chronic kidney disease." *Curr Opin Nephrol Hypertens.* 2012 Nov;21(6):635-640; Goraya N, Wesson DE. "Does correction of metabolic acidosis slow chronic kidney disease?" *Curr Opin Nephrol Hypertens.* 2013 Mar;22(2):193-7.

[2] Id.

[3] American Society of Nephrology (ASN) (2013, Nov 9). "Dietary acid load is associated with chronic kidney disease progression in elderly patients." (Abstract TH-PO243).

[4] National Kidney Foundation. Kidney Disease: Improving Global Outcomes (KDIGO) CKD Work Group. KDIGO 2012 Clinical Practice Guidelines for the Evaluation and Management of Chronic Kidney Disease. *Kidney Int., Suppl.* 2013;3:1-150.

[5] Goraya N, Simoni J, Jo CH, Wesson DE. "A comparison of treating metabolic acidosis in CKD stage 4 hypertensive kidney disease with fruits and vegetables or sodium bicarbonate." *Clin J Am Soc Nephrol.* 2013 Mar;8(3):371-81; Scilla JJ, Anderson CA. "Dietary acid load: A novel nutritional target in chronic kidney disease?" *Adv Chronic Kidney Dis.* 2013 Mar:20(2):141-9.

[6] American Society of Nephrology (ASN) (2013, Nov 9). "Fruits and vegetables or oral NaHCO3 prevent progression of kidney injury in stage 1 CKD due to hypertensive nephrology." (Abstract FR-PO816).

[7] van den Berg E, Engberink MF, Brink EJ, et al. "Dietary acid load and metabolic acidosis in renal transplant recipients." *Clin J Am Soc Nephrol.* 2012 Nov:7(11):1811-8.

Inflammation: Internal Attack

[1] Krane V, Wanner C. "Statins, inflammation, and kidney disease: inflammation in patients with CKD." *Nat Rev Nephrol.* 2011 May 31;7(7):385-97.

[2] Krishnamurthy VMR, Wei G, Baird B, et al. "High dietary fiber intake is associated with decreased Inflammation and all-cause mortality in patients with chronic kidney disease." *Kidney International.* 2012;81:300-306.

[3] Jiang L, Huang W, Liang Y, et al. "Metabolic syndrome, C-reactive protein and micro albuminuria in rural chinese population: a cross-sectional study." *BMC Nephrol.* 2013 Jun 2;14(1):118.

[4] Id.

[5] Krishnamurthy VMR, Wei G, Baird B, et al. "High dietary fiber intake is associated with decreased inflammation and all-cause mortality in patients with chronic kidney disease." *Kidney International.* 2012;81:300-306.

[6] Jiang L, Huang W, Liang Y, et al. "Metabolic syndrome, C-reactive protein and micro-albuminuria in rural chinese population: a cross-sectional study."*BMC Nephrol.* 2013 Jun 2;14(1):118; Gupta AK, Johnson WD, Johannsen D, Ravussin E. "Cardiovascular risk escalation with caloric excess." *Cardiovasc Diabetol.* 2013;12(23).

Uric Acid: Contributes to Acidosis

[1]Jalal DI, Chronchol M, Chen W, Targher G. "Uric acid as a target of therapy in CKD." *Am J Kidney Dis.* 2013;61(1):134-146.

[2]Serum uric acid treatment goal in the 2012 American College of Rheumatology Guidelines for Management of Gout.

[3]Weiner DE. "Uric acid and the kidneys: a role for urate lowering?" Discussion topic at National Kidney Foundation's 2013 Spring Clinical Meetings in Orlando, Fla., April 2-6.

[4]American College of Rheumatology (ACR) (2013 Oct 27). "Impact of urate-lowering therapy on kidney disease in people with hyperuricemia."

[5]Karalius VP, Shoham DA. "Dietary sugar and artificial sweetener intake and chronic kidney disease: a review." *Advanced Chronic Kidney Dis.* 2013 Mar;20(2):157-64.

[6]Tsai YT, Liu JP, Tu Yk, et al. "Relationship between dietary patterns and serum uric acid concentrations among ethnic Chinese adults in Taiwan." *Asia Pac J Clin Nutr.* 2012;21(2):263-70.

Be Protein Picky

[1]Goraya N, Wesson DE. "Dietary management of chronic kidney disease: protein restriction and beyond." *Curr Opin Nephrol Hypertens.* 2012 Nov;21(6):635-40.

[2]National Kidney Foundation. Kidney Disease: Inproving Global Outcomes (KDIGO), CKD Work Group. KDIGO 2012 Clinical Practice Guidelines for the Evaluation and Management of Chronic Kidney Disease. *Kidney Inter. Suppl.* 2013;3:75-76; National Kidney Foundation. KDOQITM Clinical Practice Guidelines and Clinical Practice Recommendations for Diabetes and Chronic Kidney Disease. *Am J Kidney Dis.* 49:S1-S180, 2007 (suppl 2), Guideline 5.

[3]Institute of Medicine. Dietary Reference Intakes. http://www.iom.edu/Reports/2002/Dietary-Reference-Intakes-for-Energy-Carbohydrate-Fiber-Fat-Fatty-Acids-Cholesterol-Protein-and-Amino-Acids.aspx

[4]National Kidney Foundation. KDOQITM Clinical Practice Guidelines and Clinical Practice Recommendations for Diabetes and Chronic Kidney Disease. *Am J Kidney Dis.* 49:S1-S180, 2007 (suppl 2), Guideline 5.

[5]Nutrient values throughout the book come from: U.S. Department of Agriculture, Agricultural Research Service. 2012. USDA National Nutrient Database for Standard Reference, Release 25. Nutrient Data Laboratory Home Page, http://www.ars.usda.gov/nutrientdata

[6]Moore LW, Byham-Gray LD, Parrott J, et al. "The mean dietary protein intake at different stages of chronic kidney disease is higher than current guidelines." *Kidney Int.* 2013 Apr;83(4):724-32.

[7]Wu HL, Sung JM, Kao Md, et al. "Nonprotein calorie supplement improves adherence to low-protein diet and exerts beneficial responses on renal function in chronic kidney disease." *J Ren Nutr.* 2013 Jul;23 (4):271-6.

[8]Goraya N, Wesson DE. "Dietary management of chronic kidney disease: protein restriction and beyond." *Curr Opin Nephrol Hypertens.* 2012 Nov;21(6):635-40.

[9]American Society of Nephrology (ASN) (2013 Nov 7). "Consuming more vegetable protein may help patients with chronic kidney disease live longer."

[10]Fillpowicz R, Beddhu S. "Optimal nutrition for predialysis chronic kidney disease." Adv Chronic Kidney Dis. 2013 Mar;20(2):175-80.

[11]Nezu U, Kamiyama H, Kondo Y, et al. "Effect of low-protein diet on kidney function in diabetic nephropathy: meta-analysis of randomised controlled trials." *BMU OPEN.* 2013 May 28;3(5); Garneata L, Mircescu G. "Effect of low-protein diet supplemented with keto acids on progression of chronic kidney disease." *J Ren Nutr.* 2013 May;23(3):210-3.

Those Pesky Electrolytes

[1] Centers of Disease Control and Prevention, National Center for Chronic Disease Prevention and Health Promotion. Sodium Fact Sheet. http://www.cdc.gov/Features/dsSodium/; U.S. Department of Health and Human Services, U.S. Department of Agriculture. Dietary Guidelines for Americans 2010. Washington, DC: Government Publishing Office, 2010.

[2] Id.

[3] Aburto NJ, Ziolkovka A, Hooper L, et al. "Effect of lower sodium intake on health: systematic review and meta-analyses." *BMJ*. 2013 Apr. 3;346:f1326.

[4] Forman JP, Scheven L, de Jong PE, et al. "Association between sodium intake and change in uric acid, urine albumin excretion, and the risk of developing hypertension." *Circulation*. 2012 Jun 26;125(25):3108-16.

[5] National Kidney Foundation. Kidney Disease: Improving Global Outcomes (KDIGO) CKD Work Group. KDIGO 2012 Clinical Practice Guidelines for the Evaluation and Management of Chronic Kidney Disease. *Kidney Int., Suppl.* 2013;3:78, citing Swift PA, Markandu ND, Sagnella GA, et al. "Modest salt reduction reduces blood pressure and urine protein in black hypertensives: a randomized control trial." *Hypertens*. 2005; 46:308-312.

[6] McMahon EJ, Bauer JD, Hawley CM, et al. "A randomized trial of dietary sodium restriction in CKD." *J Am Soc Nephrol*. 2013 Dec;24(12):2096-103. See also, de Brito-Ashurst I, Perry L, Sanders TA, et al. "The role of salt intake and salt sensitivity in the management of hypertension in South Asian people with chronic kidney disease: a randomized controlled study." *Heart*. 2013 Sep;99(17):1256-60.

[7] Aburto NJ, Hanson S, Gutierrez H, et al. "Effect of increased potassium intake on cardiovascular risk factors and disease: systematic review and meta-analyses." *BMJ*. 2013 Apr 3;346:f1378.

[8] U.S. Department of Health and Human Services, U.S. Department of Agriculture. Dietary Guidelines for Americans 2010. Washington, DC: Government Publishing Office, 2010.

[9] National Kidney Foundation. KDOQITM Clinical Practice Guidelines and Clinical Practice Recommendations for Diabetes and Chronic Kidney Disease. *Am J Kidney Dis*. 49:S1-S180, 2007 (suppl 2), Guideline 5.

[10] http://www.kidney.org/atoz/content/potassium.cfm.

[11] Block GA, Ix JH, Ketteler M, et al. "Phosphate homeostasis in CKD: Report of a scientific symposium sponsored by the National Kidney Foundation." *Am J Kidney Dis*. 2013 Sep;62(3):457-73.

[12] Leon JB, Sullivan CM, Sehgal AR. "Prevalence of phosphorus-containing food additives in top-selling foods in grocery stores." J Ren Nutr. 2013 Jul;23(4):265-270.

[13] Moe Sm, Zidehsarsi MP, Chambers Ma, et al. "Vegetable compared with meat dietary protein and phosphorus homeostasis in chronic kidney disease." *Clin J Am Soc Nephrol*. 2011 Feb;6(2):257-64.

[14] Shoham DA, Durazo-Arvizu R, Kramer H, et al. "Sugary soda consumption and albuminuria: results from the National Health and Nutrition Examination Survey, 1999-2004." *PLoS One*. 2008;3(10):e3431.

[15] http://www.kidney.org/atoz/content/phosphorus.cfm.

Food After Kidney Transplantation

[1] van den Berg E, Engberink MF, Brink EJ, et al. "Dietary acid load and metabolic acidosis in renal transplant recipients." *Clin J Am Nephrol*. 2012 Nov;7(11):1811-8.

[2] Id.

³U.S. Renal Data system, USRDS 2013 Annual Data Report: Atlas of Chronic Kidney Disease and End-Stage Renal Disease in the United States, National Institutes of Health, National Institute of Diabetes and Digestive and Kidney Disease, Bethesda, MD. 2013;Vol.2, Ch.7.

⁴National Kidney Foundation. KDOQITM Clinical Practice Guidelines and Clinical Practice Recommendations for Diabetes and Chronic Kidney Disease. *Am J Kidney Dis.* 49:S1-S180, 2007 (suppl 2), Guideline 5.

⁵Mangray M, Vella JP. "Hypertension after kidney transplant." *Am J Kidney Dis.* 2011;57:331.

⁶U.S. Renal Data System, USRDS 2013 Annual Data Report: Atlas of Chronic Kidney Disease and End-Stage Renal Disease in the United States, National Institutes of Health, National Institute of Diabetes and Digestive and Kidney Disease, Bethesda, MD. 2013;Vol.2, Ch.7.

⁷Bienaime F, Girard D, Anglicheau D, et al. "Vitamin D status and outcomes after renal transplantation." *J Am Soc Nephrol.* 2013 Apr;24(5):831-41.

⁸U.S. Renal Data System, USRDS 2013 Annual Data Report: Atlas of Chronic Kidney Disease and End-Stage Renal Disease in the United States, National Institutes of Health, National Institute of Diabetes and Digestive and Kidney Disease, Bethesda, MD. 2013;Vol.2, Ch.7.

Chapter 5 - Smoothie Tips

Organic Versus Conventional

¹Smith-Spangler C, Brandeau ML, Hunter GE, et al. "Are organic foods safer and healthier than conventional alternatives?: a systematic review." *Ann Intern Med.* 2012 Sep 4;157(5):348-66.

²Environmental Working Group. Executive Summary of the Environmental Working Group. http://www.ewg.org/foodnews/summary.php.

Caution With Dietary Supplements

¹Grubbs V, Plantinga LC, Tuot DS, et al. "Americans' use of dietary supplements that are potentially harmful in CKD." *Am J Kidney Dis.* 2013;61(5):739-747.

²Bjelakovic G, Gluud C. "Vitamin and mineral supplement use in relation to all-cause mortality in the Iowa Women's Health Study." *Arch Intern Med.* 2011 Oct 10;171(18):1633-4.

³Xiao Q, Murphy RA, Houston DK, et al. "Dietary supplemental calcium intake and cardiovascular disease mortality: the National Institutes of health-AARP Diet and Health Study." *Jama Intern Med.* 2013 Feb 4:1-8.

⁴Id.

⁵Dore RK. "Should healthy people take calcium and vitamin D to prevent fractures? What the US Preventative Services Task Force and others say." *Cleve Clin J Med.* 2013 Jun;80(6):341-4.

⁶U.S. Department of Agriculture and U.S. Department of Health and Human Services. *Dietary Guidelines for Americans, 2010.* 7th Edition, Washington, D.C.; U.S. Government Printing Office, December 2010. Ch.5:49.

⁷National Kidney Foundation. "Use of herbal supplements in chronic kidney disease." mwww.kidney.org/atoz/content/herbalsupp.cfm.

⁸Grubbs V, Plantinga LC, Tuot DS, et al. "Americans' use of dietary supplements that are potentially harmful in CKD." *Am J Kidney Dis.* 2013;61(5):739-747.

⁹Id.

Major Caution

¹⁰Herbland A, El Zein, Valentino R, et al. "Star fruit poisoning is potentially life-threatening in patients with moderate chronic kidney failure." *Intensive Care Med.* 2009 Aug;35(8):1459-63.

Chapter 6 - Why Smoothies?

[1] Cahill LE, Chiuve SE, Mekary RA, et al. "Prospective study of breakfast eating and incident coronary heart disease in a cohort of male US health professionals." *Circulation.* 2013 Jul 23;128(4):337-43.

[2] Fillpowicz R, Beddhu S. "Optimal nutrition for predialysis chronic kidney disease." *Adv Chronic Kidney Dis.* 2013 Mar;20(2):175-80.

[3] Id.

Part 4 - Smoothies for Most

[1] Velasquez MT, Bhathena SJ, Ranich T, et al. "Dietary flaxseed meal reduces proteinuria and ameliorates nephropathy in an animal model of type II diabetes mellitus." *Kidney Int.* 2003 Dec;64(6):2100-7.

[2] Fernandes MB, Caldas HC, Martins LR, et al. "Effects of polyunsaturated fatty acids (PUFAs) in the treatment of experimental chronic renal failure." *Int Urol Nephrol.* 2012 Oct;44(5):1571-6.

[3] Yokozawa T, Noh JS, Park CH. "Green tea polyphenols for the protection against renal damage caused by oxidative stress." *Evid Based Complement Alternat Med.* 2012;2012:845917.

[4] Cassidy A, Mukamal KJ, Liu L, et al. "High anthocyanin intake is associated with a reduced risk of myocardial infarction in young and middle-aged women." *Circulation.* 2013 Jan 15;127(4):188-96.

[5] Saafi-Ben Salah EB, El Arem A, Louedi M, et al. "Antioxidant-rich date palm fruit extract inhibits oxidative stress and nephrotoxicity induced by dimethoate in rat." *J Physiol Biochem.* 2012 Mar;68(1):47-58.

[6] Zhang Y, Neogi T, Chen C, et al. "Cherry consumption and decreased risk of recurrent gout attacks." *Arthritis Rheum.* 2012 Dec;64(12):4004-11.

[7] Lea JP. "Metabolic syndrome, CKD progression, and death: the good, the bad, and the ugly." *Clin J Am Soc Nephrol.* 2013 Jun;8(6):893-5.

[8] Nair S, O'Brien SV, Hayden K, et al. "Effect of a cooked meat meal on serum creatinine and estimated glomerular filtration rate in diabetes related kidney disease." *Diabetes Care.* 2013 Sept 23. PMID: 24062331.

[9] Schurgers LJ. "Vitamin K: key in controlling vascular calcification in chronic kidney disease."*Kidney Int.* 2013 May;83(5):782-4.

[10] Panagiotakos D. "A Mediterranean diet supplemented with olive oil or nuts reduces the incidence of major cardiovascular events in high-risk patients." *Evid Based Med.* 2013 Sept;14(3):255-63.

[11] Quirk SE, Williams LJ, O'Neil A, et al. "The association between diet quality, dietary patterns and depression in adults: a systematic review." *BMC Psychiatry.* 2013 Jun 27;13:175.

[12] Molina P, Gorriz JL, Molina MD, et al. "The effect of cholecalciferol for lowering albuminuria in chronic kidney disease: a prospective controlled study." *Nephrol Dial Transplant.* 2013 Aug 24. PMID: 23975842.

[13] Skaaby T, Husemoen LL, Plsinger C, et al. "Vitamin D status and 5-year changes in urine albumin creatinine ratio and parathyroid hormone in a general population." *Endocrine.* 2013 Oct;44(2):473-80.

[14] Vasileiou I, Katsargyris A, Theocharis S, Glaginis C. "Current clinical status on the preventive effects of cranberry consumption against urinary tract infections." *Nutr Res.* 2013 Aug;33(8):595-607.

[15] Frasseto L, Kohistadt I. "Treatment and prevention of kidney stones: an update." *Am Fam Physician.* 2011 Dec 1;84(11):1234-32.

[16] Karalius VP, Shoham DA. "Dietary sugar and artificial sweetener intake and chronic kidney disease: a review." *Adv Chronic Kidney Dis.* 2013 Mar;20(2):157-64.

[17] Reid K, Sullivan TR, Fakler P, et al. "Effect of cocoa on blood pressure." *Cochrane Database Syst Rev.* 2012 Aug 15;8:CD008893.

[18] Results presented at European Society of Hypertension (ESH) 2013 Scientific Sessions. http://www.theheart.org/article/1553207.doa.

[19] Chang A, Van Horn L, Jacobs DR Jr, et al. "Lifestyle-related factors, obesity, and incident microalbuminuria: The CARDIA study." *Am J Kidney Dis.* 2013 Aug;62(2):267-75.

[20] Eg., Mekkes MC, Weenen TC, Brummer RJ, Claassen E. "The development of probiotic treatment in obesity: a review." *Benef Microbes.* 2013 Jul 25:1-10.

[21] Corbett C, Armstrong MJ, Neuberger J. "Tobacco smoking and solid organ transplantation." *Transplantation.* 2012 Nov 27;94(10):979-87.

[22] Ruospo M, Palmer SC, Craig Jc, et al. "Prevalence and severity of oral disease in adults with chronic kidney disease: a systematic review of observational studies." *Nephrol Dial Transplant.* 2013 Sep 29. PMID: 24081863.

[23] Goraya N, Wesson DE. "Dietary management of chronic kidney disease: protein restriction and beyond." *Curr Opin Nephrol Hypertens.* 2012 Nov;21(6):635-40.

[24] Crippa G, Bosi M, Casi L, et al. "Dietary integration with Grana Padano cheese effectively reduces blood pressure in hypertensive patients." *J Hypertension.* 2012;30 (e-Supp. S):e376.

[25] Howden EJ, Leano R, Petchey W, et al. "hinEffects of exercise and lifestyle intervention on cardiovascular function in CKD." *Clin J Am Soc Nephrol.* 2013 Sep;8(9):1494-501.

[26] Moreillon JJ, Bowden RG, Deike E, et al. "The use of anti-inflammatory supplementation in patients with chronic kidney disease." *J Complement Integr Med.* 2013 Jul 1:10.

[27] Chakkera HA, Weil EJ, Pham PT, et al. "Can new-onset diabetes after kidney transplant be prevented?" *Diabetes Care.* 2013 May;36(5):1406-12.

[28] Evenepoel P, Meijers BK. "Dietary fiber and protein: nutritional therapy in chronic kidney disease and beyond." *Kidney Int.* 2012 Feb;81(3):227-9.

[29] Salmean YA, Segal MS, Langkamp-Henken B, et al. "Foods with added fiber lower serum creatinine levels in patients with chronic kidney disease." *J Ren Nutr.* 2013 Mar;23(2):e29-32.

[30] SLEEP 2013: Associated Professional Sleep Societies 27th Annual Meeting. Abstract 0808.

[31] Barzilay JI, Lovato JF, Murray AM, et al. "Albuminuria and cognitive decline in people with diabetes and normal kidney function." *Clin J Am Soc Nephrol.* 2013 Nov;8(11):1907-14. Elgen T, Chonchol M, Forsti H, Sander D. "Chronic kidney disease and cognitive impairment: a systematic review and meta-analysis." *Am J Nephrol.* 2012;35(5):474-82.

[32] Wang CJ, Grantham JJ, Wetmore JB. "The medicinal use of water in renal disease." *Kidney Int.* 2013 Jul;84(1):45-53.

[33] Chang A, Van Horn L, Jacobs DR Jr, et al. "Life-style related factors, obesity, and incident microalbuminuria: The CARDIA study." *Am J Kidney Dis.* 2013 Aug;622):267-75; Shen W, Chen H, Chen H, et al. "Obesity-related glomerulopathy: body mass index and proteinuria." *Clin J Am Soc Nephrol.* 2010 Aug;5(8):1401-1409.

[34] http://www.kidney.org/news/ekidney/august13/Spice_Up_Your_Diet_with_7_Kidney-Friendly_Seasonings.cfm.

[35] http://www.nlm.nih.gov/medlineplus/druginfo/natural/961.html.

[36] Palatty PL, Haniadka R, Valder B, et al. "Ginger in the prevention of nausea and vomiting: a review." *Crit Rev Food Sci Nutr.* 2013;53(7):659-69.

[37] Muraki L, Imamura F, Manson JE, et al. "Fruit consumption and risk of type 2 diabetes: results from three prospective longitudinal cohort studies." *BMJ.* 2013 Aug 28;347:f5001.

[38] Chang A, Batch BC, McGuire, et al. "Association of a reduction in central obesity and phosphorus intake with changes in urinary albumin excretion: The PREMIER Study." *Am J Kidney Dis.* 2013 Nov;62(5):900-7.

[39] Levine GN, Allen K, Braun LT. "Pet ownership and cardiovascular risk: a scientific statement from the American Heart Association." *Circulation.* 2013 Jun 11;127(23):2353-63.

[40] Misurac JM, Knoderer CA, Leiser JD, et al. "Non-steroidal anti-inflammatory drugs are an important cause of acute kidney injury in children." *Pediatrics.* 2013 Jun;162(6):1153-9.

[41] Verneuil L, Varna M, Ratajczak P, et al. "Human skin carcinoma arising from kidney transplant-derived tumor cells." *J Clin Invest.* 2013 Sep 3;123(9):3797-801.

[42] Saw CL, Huang MT, Liu Y, et al. "Impact of Nrf2 on UVB-induced skin inflammation/photoprotection and photoprotective effect of sulforaphane." *Mol Carcinog.* 2011 Jun;50(6):479-86.

[43] Ghosh SM, Kapil V, Fuentes-Calco I, et al. "Enhanced vasodilator activity of nitrate in hypertension: critical role of erthrocytic xanthine oxidoreductase and translational potential." *Hypertension.* 2013 May;61(5):1091-102.

[44] Waheed A, Ludtmann MRH, Pakes N, et al. "Naringenin inhibits the growth of Dictyostelium and MDCK-derived cysts in a polycystin-2 (TRPP2)-dependent manner." Br J Pharmacol. 2013 Oct 3. PMID: 24116661.

[45] Eg., Odegaard AO, Jacobs DR Jr, Steffen LM, et al. "Breakfast frequency and development of metabolic risk." *Diabetes Care.* 2013 Oct;36(10):3100-6.

[46] Muntner P, Judd SE, Gao L, et al. "Cardiovascular risk factors in CKD associate with both ESRD and mortality." *J Am Soc Nephrol.* 2013 Jun;24(7):1159-65.

[47] Larsson SC, Virtamo J, Wolk A. "Dairy consumption and risk of stroke in Swedish women and men." *Stroke.* 2012 Jul;43(7):1775-80.

[48] Howell AB, D'Souza DH. "The pomegranate: effects on bacteria and viruses that influence human health." *Evid Based Complement Alternat Med.* 2013;2013:606212.

[49] Muraki I, Imamura F, Manson Je, et al. "Fruit consumption and risk of type 2 diabetes: results from three prospective longitudinal cohort studies." *BMJ.* 2013 Aug 28;347:f5001.

[50] Murapa P, Dai J, Chung M, et al. "Anthocyanin-rich fractions of blackberry extracts reduce UV-induced free radicals and oxidative in keratinocytes." *Phytotherapy Research.* 2012 Jan;26(1):106-112.

[51] van den Berg E, Engberink MF, Brink EJ, et al. "Dietary acid load and metabolic acidosis in renal transplant recipients." *Clin J am Soc Nephrol.* 2012 Nov;7(11):1811-8.

[52] Goraya N, Simoni J, Jo CH, Wesson DE. "A comparison of treating metabolic acidosis in CKD stage 4 hypertensive kidney disease with fruits and vegetables or sodium bicarbonate." *Clin J Am Soc Nephrol.* 2013 Mar;8(3):371-81.

Part 5 - Smoothies with Lower Potassium and Phosphorus

[1] Olyaei A, Steffl JL, Maclaughlan J, et al. "HMG-CoA reductase inhibitors in chronic kidney disease." *Am J Cardiovasc Drugs.* 2013 Dec;13(6):385-98.

[2] Allen RW, Schwartzman E, Baker WL, et al. "Cinnamon use in type 2 diabetes: an updated systematic review and meta-analysis." *Ann Fam Med.* 2013 Sept-Oct;11(5):452-459.

[3] Haniadka R, Saldanha E, Sunita V, et al. "A review of the gastroprotective effects of ginger (Zingiber officinale Roscoe)." *Food Funct.* 2013 Jun;4(6):845-55.

[4] Olyaei A, Steffl J, MacLaughlan M, et al. "HMG-Co A reductase inhibitors in chronic kidney disease." *Am J Cardiovasc Drugs.* 2013 Dec;13(6);385-98.

[5] Jennings A, Welch AA, Fairweather-Tait SJ, et al. "Higher anthocyanin intake is associated with lower arterial stiffness and central blood pressure in women." *Am J Clin Nutr.* 2012 Oct;96(4):781-8.

[6]Kanasaki K, Kitada M, Kanasaki M, Koya D. "The biological consequences of obesity on the kidney." *Nephrol Dial Transplant.* 2013 Nov;28 Suppl 4:iv1-iv7.

[7]Nguyen HT, Bertoni AG, Nettleton Ja, et al. "DASH eating pattern is associated with favorable left ventricular function in the multi-ethnic study of atherosclerosis." *J Am Coll Nutr.* 2012 Dec;31(6):401-7.

[8]Larijani VN, Ahmadi N, Zeb I, et al. "Beneficial effects of aged garlic extract and coenzyme Q10 on vascular elasticity and endothelial function: the FAITH randomized clinical trial." *Nutrition.* 2013 Jan;29(1):71-5.

[9]http://www.ncbi.nlm.nih.gov/pmc/articles/PMC2515569/.

[10]Liu B, Mao Q, Wang X, et al. "Cruciferous vegetables consumption and risk of renal cell carcinoma: a meta-analysis." *Nutr Cancer.* 2013;65(5):668-76.

[11]Yang J, Xiao YY. "Grape phytochemicals and associated health benefits." *Crit Rev Food Sci Nutr.* 2013;53(11):1202-25.

[12]Muraki I, Imamura F, Manson JE, et al. "Fruit consumption and risk of type 2 diabetes: results from three prospective longitudinal cohort studies." *BMJ.* 2013 Aug 28;347.

[13]Connery, G. C. (2013). "Curbing dietary fructose intake may be effective in decreasing elevated uric acid levels in renal disease patients." Renal & Urology News, Vol. 12 (Issue 9), p.24.

[14]Jun M, Venkataraman V, Razavian M, et al. "Antioxidants for chronic kidney disease." *Cochrane Database Syst Rev.* 2012 Oct 17;10:CD008176.

[15]Ferraro PM, Taylor EN, Eisner BH, et al. "History of kidney stones and the risk of coronary heart disease." *JAMA.* 2013 Jul 24;310(4):408-15.

[16]Eg., Correa F, Buelna-Chontal M, Hernandez-Resendiz, et al. "Curcumin maintains cardiac and mitochondrial function in chronic kidney disease." *Free Radic Biol Med.* 2013 Mar 30;61C:119-129.

[17]Swithers SE. "Artificial sweeteners produce the counterintuitive effect of inducing metabolic derangements." *Trends Endocrinol Metab.* 2013 Sep;24(9):431-41.

[18]Lin J, Curhan GC. "Associations of sugar and artificially sweetened soda with albuminuria and kidney function decline." *Clin J Am Nephrol.* 2011 Jan;6(1):160-6.

[19]Moe SM, Zidehsarai MP, Chambers MA, et al. "Vegetarian compared with meat dietary protein source and phosphorus homeostasis in chronic kidney disease." *Clin J Am Soc Nephrol.* 2011 Feb;6(2):257-64.

[20]Steiber, A. (2011, December). "Soy protein may benefit kidney disease patients." *Renal & Urology News.* Vol. 10, Issue 12.

Part 6 - Smoothies For Dialysis

[1]Stein J. (2013 Aug). Dietary Phosphorus Restriction Tough. *Renal & Urology News.* Vol.12, Issue 8, p.13.

[2]Vasquez k, et al. "Treatment of vitamin deficiency/insufficiency with ergo-calciferol is associated with reduced vascular access dysfunction in chronic hemodialysis patients with type 2 diabetes." *NKF* 2013; Abstract 108.

[3]Lemos JR, Alencastro MG, Konrath AV, et al. "Flaxseed oil supplemen-tation decreases C-reactive protein levels in chronic hemodialysis patients." *Nutr Res.* 2012 Dec;32(12):921-7.

[4]Shema-Didi L, Sela S, Ore L, et al. "One year of pomegranate juice intake decreases oxidative stress, inflammation, incidence of infections in hemodialysis patients: a randomized placebo-controlled trial." *Free Radic Biol Med.* 2012 Jul 15:53(2):297-304.

[5]Farhat G, Drummond S, Fyfe L, Al-Dujaili EA. "Dark chocolate: An obesity paradox or a culprit for weight gain?" *Phytother Res.* 2013 Sept 2. PMID: 24000103.

[6]Palatty PL, Haniadka R, Valder B, et al. "Ginger in the prevention of nausea and vomiting: a review." *Crit Rev Food Sci Nutr.* 2013;53(7):659-69.

[7] Giannaki CD, Hadjigeorgiou GM, Karatzaferi C, et al. "A single-blind randomized controlled trial to evaluate the effect of 6 months of progressive aerobic exercise training in patients with uraemic restless legs syndrome." *Nephrol Dial Transplant*. 2013 Nov;28(11):2834-40.

[8] Bao Y, Han J, Hu FB, et al. "Association of nut consumption with total and cause-specific mortality." *N Engl J Med*. 2013 Nov 21;369(21):2001-11.

[9] Kuhlmann U, Becker HF, Birkhahn M, et al. "Sleep-apnea in patients with end-stage renal disease and objective results." *Clin Nephrol*. 2000 Jun;53(6):460-6.

[10] Harley KT, Streja E, Rhee CM, et al. "Nephrologist caseload and hemodialysis survival in an urban cohort." *J Am Soc Nephrol*. 2013 Oct;24(10):1678-87.

[11] Assini JM, Mulvihill EE, Huff MW. "Citrus flavonoids and lipid metabolism." *Curr Opin Lipidol*. 2013 Feb;24(1):34-40.

[12] Eg., Figueroa A, Wong A, Hooshmand S, Sanchez-Gonzalez MA. "Effects of watermelon supplementation on arterial stiffness and wave reflection amplitude in postmenopausal women." *Menopause*. 2013 May;20(5):573-7.

[13] Preljevic VT, Osthus TB, Os I, et al. "Anxiety and depressive disorders in dialysis patients: association to health-related quality of life and mortality." *Gen Hosp Psychiatry*. 2013 Nov-Dec;35(6):619-24.

[14] Raimann JG, Levin NW, Craig RG, et al. "Is vitamin C intake too low in dialysis patients?" *Semin Dial*. 2013 Jan-Feb;26(1):1-5.

[15] Siervo M, Lai J, Ogbonmwan I, Mathers JC. "Inorganic nitrate and beetroot juice supplementation reduces blood pressure in adults: a systematic review and meta-analysis." *J Nutr*. 2013 Jun;143(6):818-26.

[16] Rautiainen S, Levitan EB, Orsini N, et al. "Total antioxidant capacity from diet and risk of myocardial infarction: a prospective cohort of women." *Am J Med*. 2012 Oct;125(10):974-80.

[17] Prasad N, Sinha A, Gupta A, et al. "Effect of metabolic syndrome on clinical outcomes of non diabetic peritoneal dialysis patients." *Nephrology (Carlton)*. 2013 Oct;18(10):657-64.

[18] West C. "Is it time for a new renal diet? Reevaluating the role of plant-based foods in the dialysis diet." *Nephrol News Issues*. 2012 Sept;26(10):21-2.

[19] Zhao S, Bomser J, Joseph EL, et al. "Intake of apples or apple poly-phenols decrease plasma values for oxidized low-density lipoprotein/beta2-glycoprotein I complex." *J Func Foods*. 2013 Jan;5(1):493-497.

[20] Afsar B. "The relation between internet and social media use and the demographic and clinical parameters, quality of life, depression, cognitive function and sleep quality in hemodialysis patients: Social media and hemodialysis." *Gen Hosp Psychiatry*. 2013 Nov-Dec;35(6):625-30.

[21] Eg., Ikizier TA, Cano NJ, Franch H, et al. "Prevention and treatment of protein energy wasting in chronic kidney disease patients: a consensus statement by the International Society of Renal Nutrition and Metabolism." *Kidney Int*. 2013 Dec;84(6):1096-107.

Index Page 1

Acai-Berry Smoothie 107
acidosis 39-42
added sugar 17, 61
aging and kidneys 8
albumin 5
albuminuria 6
Amy's Wacky Shake 117
anemia 4
Anti-Inflammatory Snack .. 104
Antioxidant Heart Power ... 161
antioxidants 32
"A" Power 119
atherosclerosis 21
Ben's Fruit Creation 98
Berries for Pressure Relief . 131
Berry-Orange Inflammation Fighter 148
Blackberry Sun Shield 123
bladder. 3
Blood Pressure Easer 157
Blood Pressure Magic 102
Bloody Mary for Health 103
Blueberry Cheesecake 149
Blueberry-Peach Tummy Soother 152
Blueberry Starter 147
calcitriol 4, 55
calcium 53
carotenoids 34
Cherries + Fiber 81
Cherry-Berry Cheesecake .. 166
cholesterol 20
chronic inflammation 43
chronic kidney disease (CKD). 5
Clara's Fruit 'n' Veggies 91

Cough and Sore Throat Soother 156
C-reactive protein 44
creatinine 6
DASH 13, 29
Dates to the Rescue 84
diabetes 11
Diabetes Ammunition 137
Diabetes Relief 122
diabetic nephropathy 12
diastolic 14
Drinkable Sunscreen 115
Easing Hypertension 160
Echoes of Apple Pie 164
electrolytes 48
end stage renal disease (ESRD) 5
erythropoietin 4
estimated GFR 5
Eva's Pink Shake 125
Experimenting with Kale 88
fats 20
fiber 35-37
Fiber Power 106
Fig-Quinoa Breakfast 118
Fitting in a Power Vege 142
free radicals 32
fructose 17
Fun with Watermelon 99
glomeruli 3
glomerulus 3
glucosinolates 34
Going Chinese 135
Green De-Stresser 105
Green Super Shake 114
Green Tea + Peaches 82

heart and kidneys 8
Heart Blush 150
herbs 69
high blood pressure 13
high density lipoprotein 21
hyperkalemia 50
hyperlipidemia 22
hypertension 13
hyperuricemia 44
inflammation 42
insoluble 35
insulin resistance 12
Jack's Orange Dreamsicle 97
Jennifer's Drinkable Pumpkin Pie 132
Jennifer's Kidney Balm 115
juicing 66
Kidney Aid 101 109
kidney failure 5
kidney function 7
kidney transplant 54-57
Kit's Indian/Thai Inspiration 89
Life's Simple 7 9
limonoids 34
lipid levels 22
lipoproteins 21
Live Long and Prosper 139
low density lipoprotein, ... 21
lycopene 34
Memory Smoothie 108
metabolic acidosis 39
metabolic syndrome 16
mono-or polyunsaturated 21
Nausea Buster 130
Nausea Easer 111
nephrons 3
obesity 15, 19

omega-3 fatty acids 21
omega-6 fatty acids 22
Orange Sherbet with a Healing Plus 162
organic foods 67
oxidative stress 33
Peaches & Cream 158
Peach Milkshake for "D" 92
Pear-Hemp Shake 125
Pear-Peach-Mango Tango . 110
Pear + Pineapple 86
Pear-Seeds-Pineapple 154
pH scale 39
phenols and polyphenols 35
phosphorus 52-53
phytochemicals 33, 34
Pineapple and Beets 116
Plum Pudding 120
Pom Power 121
potassium 49-51
protein 44, 45, 60, 71
proteinuria 6
Pumpkin + Banana 94
Red Velvet Chocolate Delight
 151
renal diet 31
renin 4
Rice Pudding 153
Salad in a Glass 96
salt 47-48
saturated fatty acids 21
Simply Blueberries 100
Snack for Lower BP 136
sodium 47-48
soluble 35
Soy and Sage Power 143
Soy-Apricot-Date Delight . 113

Spencer's Almond-Cherry Attack 85
starfruit 71
Strawberry Shake 165
Strawberry-Watermelon Mojito 83
Sully's Virgin Pina Colada .. 87
supplements 68
Swigging Salad 134
systolic 14
Taste of Turmeric 141
Touch of Fig 155
Touch of Green 129
Touch of Thyme 90
transplant recipients 42
triglycerides. 21
Tropical Delight 138
unsaturated fatty acids 21
urea 3, 46
uric acid 43
UTI and Stone Aid 93
UTI and Stone Defense 140
Vicki's Berry Blast 112
Valentine Smoothie 95
Veggie Salad Punch 163
Vitamin C Daily Dose 159
Vitamin C Delight 133
water 59

Made in the USA
San Bernardino, CA
14 March 2014